HAIRCOLORING
IN PLAIN ENGLISH

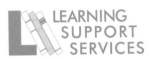

HAIRCOLORING
IN PLAIN ENGLISH

by Roxy A. Warren

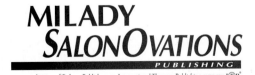

MILADY
SalonOvations
PUBLISHING

a division of Delmar Publishers, an International Thomson Publishing company I(T)P®

3 Columbia Circle, P.O. Box 12519 • Albany, New York 12212-2519

NOTICE TO THE READER

Cover Design: Suzanne Nelson
Cover Photos Courtesy of: Brian and Sandra Smith (upper left), Epic the Salon (lower left), and Koger-LaPrairie for Salon JKL (lower right)

Milady Staff
Acquisitions Editor: Pamela Lappies
Developmental Editor: Joseph Miranda
Project Editor: NancyJean Downey
Production Manager: Brian Yacur
Production and Art/Design Coordinator: Suzanne Nelson

COPYRIGHT © 1999
Milady Publishing
(a division of Delmar Publishers)
an International Thomson Publishing company

Printed in the United States of America
Printed and distributed simultaneously in Canada

For more information, contact:
Milady/SalonOvations Publishing
3 Columbia Circle , Box 12519
Albany, New York 12212-2519

3 4 5 6 7 8 9 10 QPD 03

Library of Congress Cataloging-in-Publication Data

Warren, Roxy A.
    Haircoloring in plain english / by Roxy A. Warren.
       p.   cm.
    Includes bibliographical references and index.
    ISBN: 1-56253-357-6
    1. Hair—Dyeing and bleaching.   I. Title.
TT973.W37   1998   98-3966
646.7'24—dc21   CIP

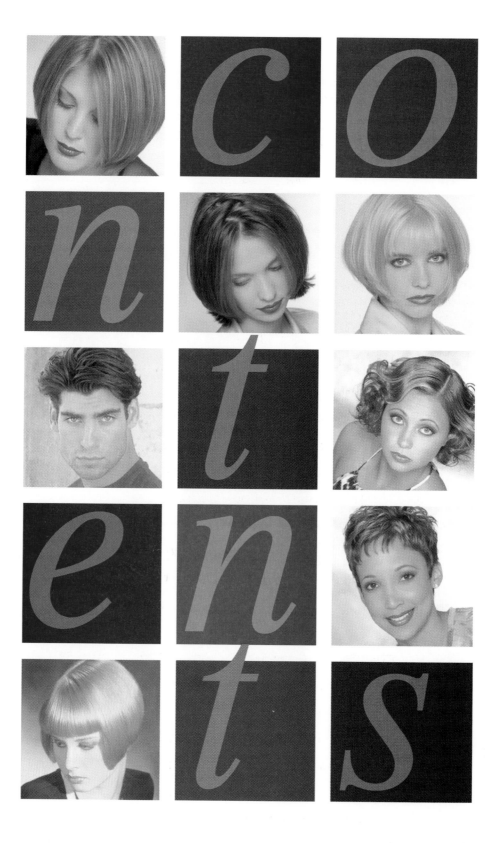

contents

Dedication

For my husband, Dr. John V. Aliff

introduction

Excellent color skills are a necessity—not a plus, but a must. It doesn't matter where your salon is or what your target market is—your clients want you to color their hair and you have to know how.

This book was written at the request of a friend of mine, the owner of an upscale salon in a highly competitive, metropolitan market. She needed a generic color manual to train incoming employees and to serve as a reference for existing staff—stylists of all levels of experience—to ensure that everyone knew haircoloring. When she could not find such a book, she asked me to write this one.

At its essence, this is a formulation book. It is also a color theory book and a corrective haircoloring book, written from a stylist's point of view rather than by a manufacturer, and it contains not just one person's ideas, but many stylists' ideas. Throughout are pointers and technical notes on a great many topics within the realm of salon haircoloring. The last unit of the book consists of marketing and management information derived from the experiences of salon owners and my experience as a training manager.

The Importance of Haircoloring Services

Roughly half of the U.S. population is age 35 or older.[1] Clients are aging, graying, and requesting color. But there's so much more to it than that.

Artificial haircoloring has come of age. It is accepted and appreciated as a personal accessory. Coloring your hair is considered good grooming, part of taking care of yourself,

not vanity or luxury. And it's just daring enough and important enough to require professional assistance.

Great haircoloring is transforming. It makes the wearer feel good. It changes her (or him) inside and out. Color is every bit as image-enhancing and confidence-boosting as the right haircut or make-up. A color client shakes her hair on the way out the salon door and can't get enough of herself in the mirror—just like cut clients.

Gregory Carlyle, accomplished stylist, salon owner and platform artist, says, "We need to recognize that haircoloring is not only for covering gray, but also for creating additional body and shine in the hair, and for creating *change* for the client—for fashion reasons as well as practical reasons. The young people present a tremendous market."

Earn a living in the salon for a while, and you quickly learn to appreciate color! Color is profitable, and color makes clients loyal like nothing else can.

A client may get a trim elsewhere, or even a perm, but not her retouch. Michele Dubourdieu, a colorist who has developed numerous haircoloring products and trained innumerable colorists, says, "When a color client goes on a vacation, her colorist is the last person she sees before she leaves and the first person she sees when she gets back—the appointment is already made." Clients depend most on their stylists when it comes to color.

A reputation as a good haircolorist practically ensures a strong and steady clientele. Conversely, a stylist who is not willing nor able to do good color services will have difficulty retaining clients (unless the salon is specialized), simply because there are too many people who need or want color. Clients will

---

1 *Statistical Abstract of the United States, Washington, DC: US Bureau of the Census, 1993; p.17.*

find someone to do their color the way they want it, and eventually that salon will be cutting and perming them, too.

For profitability, it is hard to beat color! Haircoloring services help maximize the stylist's time in the salon. Application time for color is relatively brief. And while the color processes, the stylist can perform another service. The dollar return on the stylist's time is higher for haircoloring than almost any other service. Furthermore, color clients average more salon visits per year than any other group (they come more often)—and spend more money at the salon yearly (they buy more services and products).

There are greater opportunities in color today, and more challenges, too. Advances in products have helped to make us better colorists. Our dispensaries are packed with products of tremendous quality and variety, and we have to know what to do with them. Training is also more available today; more stylists understand color and do it well. And clients have more options and higher expectations than ever before—they know the difference between mediocre and great haircoloring and expect value for their dollar.

Becoming a Good Haircolorist

If you are a good haircolorist, it is because you have done plenty of color. You have learned from your successes and your failures. You try new products and techniques. You have never stopped reading and going to classes, because you know there is always something else to learn, even if it is just relearning something you used to know.

If you are not yet an expert colorist, then this is my advice: act like one. You have heard the phrase, "fake it until you make it." Some take exception to this attitude, but if we were all to wait until we were experts to begin earning a living, no one would ever become an expert. There would be no experts, because we would all starve somewhere along the way. Talent travels a long, winding road to expertise. It is a journey that never really ends, and it has to start somewhere. Let's face it: Experience is the best teacher; the trick is in having many more good than bad experiences. And that's where emulating success comes in. Do what the experts do! Set yourself up to succeed.

Read everything you can find about color. Study and follow manufacturer's directions. Make it your purpose to know every detail about the products you use. Whenever you get a chance to go to a color class, go!

Never let a chance to color hair get away from you. Make opportunities to do color. Carlos Valenzuela once had a banner in his exceptional, Phoenix, Arizona, school that read: "If it moves, color it!" The more you do, the more you will know.

Accept your mistakes, understand them, and remember them. Remember all the perfect results, too!

Learn from the stylists around you. (Let somebody else make a few of the mistakes.)

Be versatile—try it all! (Maybe on a mannequin the first time, or a very good friend.)

Any stylist reading these words has what it takes to do great haircoloring. If you want to, you can be an excellent colorist. Shawn Clary, a stylist and talented educator from Memphis, Tennessee, used to say something like this, "A good colorist doesn't have some kind of special magic that no one else has. Haircoloring isn't magic! Haircoloring is learned." What good colorists have is knowledge—information. Fundamentally, what good colorists know is basic color theory. Good color results are due to knowledge—not magic, luck, or genius.

The greatest obstacle aspiring colorists face is the "FUD" factor: Fear, Uncertainty, and Doubt. There isn't a hairdresser alive who hasn't had a case of nerves over a color service and said prayers in the dispensary!

Fear comes from lack of knowledge. The fear that you and I feel is fear of the unknown, "Will it turn out? Does this really work? Will it look good on her?" Confidence comes from knowledge and experience; knowledge makes fear go away. To develop confidence, you must study, and you must do color services to prove to yourself that what you have read or heard really is true. Seeing color theory in action will make you a believer; it will take away your doubt and give you courage—so put forth the effort to study, then get out on a limb and do plenty of color services!

The more color you do, the more color you will do! When you send color clients out the door, more come knocking. So, if you want to do more color, then *do more color!* Salon owner, if you want your salon to be a "color" salon, hire stylists who like to do color.

A Good Haircolorist...

- **Knows and applies basic color principles. These are the universal concepts heard over and over again, because they are true regardless of brand.**
- **Reads manufacturers' literature. Printed materials from manufacturers are very reliable, designed only to increase your success.**

Read and heed all directions, especially when getting to know a new product.
- **Communicates carefully with clients. Inadequate communication is the number one cause for corrective haircoloring. Avoid re-do's by establishing in advance what the client needs and wants.**
- **Recommends color services. If a client isn't wearing haircoloring, then she probably doesn't know what's available or what's advisable—and she won't know, until you tell her (or until your competition tells her). "It is not enough to suggest," says stylist and industry leader** John Fail, **"you must recommend."**
- **Formulates simply. It very often takes only one tube, or one bottle, to make a beautiful color. (The manufacturer wouldn't put those pigments together in a single tube if they didn't make a pretty color!) Moreover, using one color at a time is the only way to train your eye to a new color line. If you always mix, you won't know where the tone or depth comes from.**
- **Formulates and applies color methodically. The way to get consistently good results is to use good methods consistently. This is true of more than just**

color; it is true of cutting, perming, and every other service.

• **Learns from every color done.** The most valuable thing anyone ever told me about haircoloring came from Michele Dubourdieu, European Technical Director for a color company based in Great Britain. She teaches colorists to study the hair before the color goes on, and then study it again when the service is complete. "Really inspect the hair," she says, "memorize what you see, before and after." When you do this, you teach your eyes to see color—to distinguish even slight variations in tone or level.

• **Learns from colleagues!** This includes classes, books, magazines, professional meetings, shows, and any other opportunities to observe another's work.

The author welcomes your comments, suggestions, and queries. Please write to P.O. Box 506, Auburn, GA 30011.

about the title

I read *Economics in Plain English,* by Leonard Silk, in 1979, while taking a college economics course. (I was also in cosmetology school at the time.) Silk's book sounded like what I needed; maybe I could learn something about economics—this intimidating subject— from someone who spoke on my level. It helped; I got an "A" in the course.

Leonard Silk, himself a practicing economist, helped me to understand economics in a way that neither my professor nor my textbook could. His simplicity, and his enthusiasm for his subject, made the information meaningful to me. It is my hope that this book, written by a practitioner of haircoloring, will make a difference in your understanding of color and in your professional life.

Silk wrote that "to economize is to choose"[1]—to choose how to use scarce resources, including personal resources, like time, for the best return. When you learn from another person's experiences, that's good economy. Books are an economical way to learn.

In writing this book, I have tried to present basic haircoloring information as simply as possible, including only and all the most vital subjects, properly researched and in clear language. I hope you find it an interesting and valuable reference.

---

1 Silk, L., Economics in Plain English *(New York, NY: Simon and Schuster, 1978), p. 57.*

a c k n o w l e d g m e n t s

This book was written in community with fellow colorists, salon owners, cosmetic chemists and others. It is the product of the experiences and wisdom of many people. It was initiated at the suggestion of my good friend, Atlanta salon owner and hairdresser's hairdresser, Kathryn Pilczuk. Thank you, Kathryn.

There are many people who were instrumental in the writing of this book and to whom I am most grateful. I owe a special debt of gratitude to the four people who reviewed the manuscript at various stages of imperfection, challenging, correcting and animating my thinking: three wonderful stylists, Andrew Covelluzzi, John Fail, and Dwight Miller, and cosmetic chemist, Dr. Leszek Wolfram. Each of these generous individuals read all or part of the book at different times and offered his expert opinion; each has my enduring thanks.

Leszek Wolfram is a most accomplished and respected cosmetic chemist—author of more than seventy articles published in international and American science journals, recepient of prestigious research awards—besides being very gracious. At one time he was V.P. of Research at the world's second largest haircoloring company; now he travels the globe wherever chemistry calls. Dr. Wolfram gave freely of his time, answering questions and reviewing scientific passages; thank you, Dr. Wolfram.

John Fail, a hairdresser who has done nearly everything in the hair business there is to do (and done it well), has been a mentor to me and to many other fortunate stylists. His lessons fill these pages. Both he and Andrew Covelluzzi, a respected colorist and owner of a salon in Salem, Massachusetts, suggested the addition of key topics. Thank you, John, and thank you, Andrew.

Dwight Miller has been doing good things in our industry for more than 30 years. He has been artistic director for several major companies, authored a haircutting book, created many techniques and trends, and now presides over his own product company. Dwight kindly read an early draft of this book and offered comments that spurred research and influenced the general tone of the book; thank you, Dwight.

I extend special thanks, also, to each of the extraordinary stylists who contributed experiences and perspectives: Kenneth Anders, Frank Barrett, Steven Brooks, Michael Burton, Billie Capps, Gregory Carlyle, Vickie Chepus, Delores Davis, Dhaniel Doud, Bruce du Bois, Jaime Escobedo, Bobby and Voula Fairbanks, Eric Fisher, Andre Galuska, Belinda and Frank Gambuzza, Jerry Gordon, Charles Gregory, Darleen Hakola, John Hickox, Bobby J. Hunt, Lili Jakel, Sam Lapin, Max Matteson, Robert Austin Miller, Reginald Mitchell, LeeAnn Nelbach, Kay Nielsen, Andre Nizetich, Edie Noppenberger, Jason Peller, Jerry Poer, David Pressley, Stacie Sanderford, Joe Santy, Ruth Sinclair, John Sloan, Judith Stephens, Sandie Talkington, Robin Todd, Susan and Albert Trombley, Clay Wilson, and Norman Zapien. All these people are heroes of hairdressing and deserve to have their stories told in a way that space here just doesn't allow. Thank you everyone.

My special thanks also to Dr. David Cannell, highly regarded cosmetic chemist and V.P. of Research at one of the world's most influential salon product companies, who patiently answered questions and sent a stack of information, complete with lab swatches. Thank you, Dr. Cannell.

Margee Bright-Ragland, Dr. John Corbett, Mark Foley, Leland Hirsch, Lee Hoffman,

Robin LeVan, Robert Oppenheim, Bill Peplow, Roy Peters, Vern Silberman, Dane Smith and Dr. Eric Warren, distinguished professionals all, thank you very much for your time, help, and unique information.

To the late, much loved Arnold (Arnie) Miller, whose memory continues to inspire so many of us, thank you from the bottom of my heart. Thanks also to Shawn Clary, Pat Johnson, and Penny Parker.

Michele Dubourdieu, Fugi Escobedo, Carole Lyden Smith and Carlos Valenzuela— thank you for your example and the loan of a few of your words.

D.J. Tenbrink, teacher, example, friend: thank you always.

The publisher and I thank the color companies that generously provided implements and products for use as illustrators' models: ArTec, Aveda, Clairol, Farouk Systems, Framesi, Goldwell, Matrix and Redken. Our thanks also to Metropolis (importer of Matador gloves), and Takara Belmont and Yu's International (makers of color processing machines).

Our thanks to the stylists and salons who provided photographs or business materials used in illustrations: George Alderete and Sculpt Salon, Dennis and Sylvia Gebhart, Gene Juarez Salons, Arlene Klass-Davidson and Epic the Salon, Janie Koger-LaPrairie and Ken LaPrairie, DonPaul and Dawnel LeBlanc and Paris Parker Salon and Spa, Lisa Learmonth and Studio Savvy, Melissa D. Monh and Fantastic Sams, Nena Perez, Piero Salon, Brigitte Pipkin, Pon Saradeth and Pon International, Saverio Ravenda and Julian Hans Salon, Linda Ramos, Brian and Sandra Smith, and Hugo/Heather Solana.

The publisher would like to thank Kelly Taggert and Purely Visual for their assistance in obtaining art. Their efforts and talent are greatly appreciated.

The publisher would like to thank the following professionals who reviewed this manuscript: Darleen Hakola, Portland, Oregon; Colleen Hennessey, Stamford, Connecticut; Liki Jakel, Toronto, Canada; and Lois Leytem, Dubuque, Iowa.

part one

1

basic haircoloring theory

Basic haircoloring theory is that body of information that does not vary from color company to color company. These are the universal concepts that always apply, no matter what brand of haircoloring is used.

From the very first haircoloring lesson in cosmetology school, these are the laws that are taught, over and over, whenever haircoloring is taught. A working understanding of basic theory is a prerequisite for the development of good formulation and application skills. And, as important as it is, this information does not have to be complicated. It does not have to be hard to understand.

The technical background of a colorist includes three basic subjects: color, hair, and haircoloring products. This is what happens when hair is colored:

Natural color + the haircoloring formula = the color result

(OR)

Natural pigment + dyestuff + developer
= the color result

(OR)

Lightened natural pigment + artificial pigment
= the color result.

To achieve a desired color result, you must understand the interaction of haircoloring chemicals and the hair fiber. You must understand the hair you are coloring (natural pigment and structural characteristics), the haircoloring product you are using (categories of haircoloring products and specific product knowledge), and what happens when the two intersect (The Law of Color).

This unit is divided into three chapters. Chapter One, Color Principles, deals with the characteristics and nature of color itself. Chapter Two, Hair Structure and Natural Pigment, describes the basic architecture of hair, the study of hair melanin, and the effect of texture and porosity. Chapter Three, Categories of Haircoloring Products, explains the characteristics, general chemistry, and uses of the product categories.

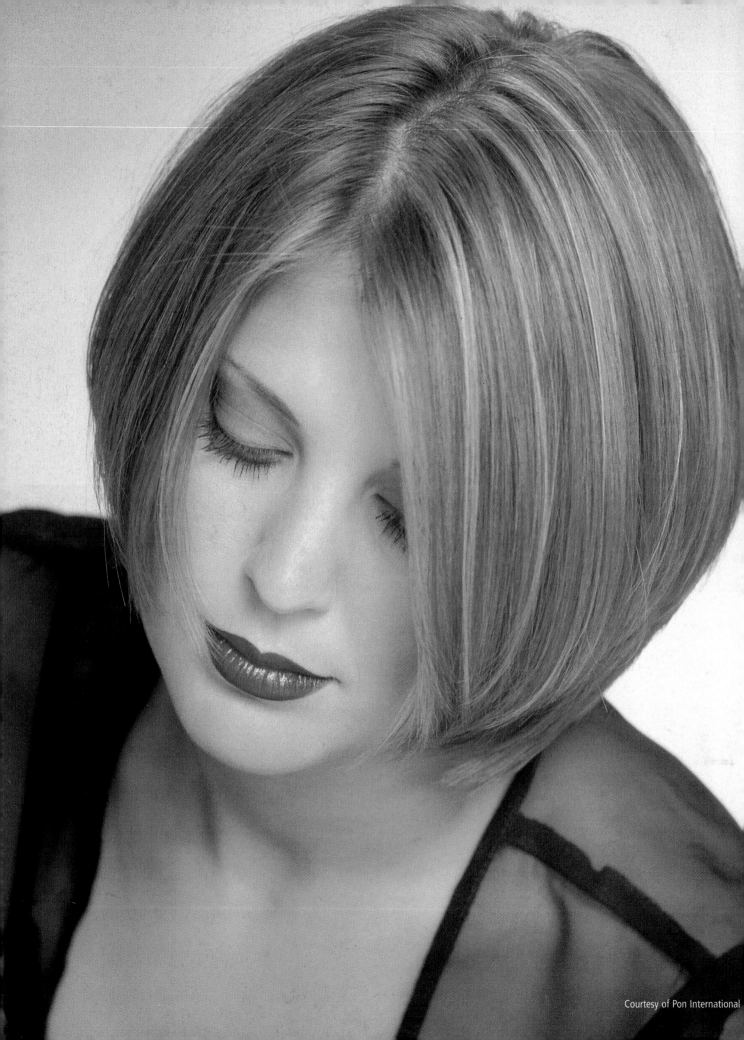

color principles

Color, as a study in itself, spills into many disciplines: art principles pertaining to color, the physics of light, the chemistry of pigments, optical effects (the effect of one color beside another, or of "aftercolors," for examples), the psychology of color. It is a study you will return to all your professional life because it is foundational to haircoloring, and because it is too sprawling a subject to get it all at one go-through.

To formulate haircoloring, you must have a *basic* understanding of color: the characteristics of color (especially level, tone, and intensity) and basic color wheel theory (especially the law of contracting colors). You don't have to become a chemist or physicist to color hair well! But after you learn the basics you will probably want to know more, because it is such an intriguing subject, and because knowing more will help you to *see* color—to distinguish even minor variations in tone or level, and to see which colors suit clients best.

Andrew Covelluzzi

master colorist and owner of
Andrew Michaels Hair Studios in
Salem, Massachusetts:

"Creativity begins with understanding the basics. You have to
understand the basics of color
to get creative with it . . .
"Understanding color gave me
a deeper sense of accomplishing
change. Understanding how color
could compliment, contrast, or
augment—why did certain shades
look better, and what were my
eyes really seeing? The excite-
ment was seeing these changes."

WHAT IS COLOR?

Color is light, pigment, and perception. It is a physical, chemical, optical, and psychological phenomenon. **Color** is the product of:

1. **available light,**
2. **the pigmentation and surface properties of things, and**
3. **the visual acuity of the onlooker.**

How Color Occurs

We say that pigments give objects color—for example, melanin gives color to skin and hair, and chlorophyll makes grass green—but pigments themselves are not "colored." Rather, pigments cause objects to reflect or absorb light a certain way, and reflected light is what we interpret as color. **Pigments** are part of the chemical structure of plants, animals, and objects. *Pigments impart color by modifying light,* absorbing part of it and reflecting the rest. What is reflected is what the eye sees, and what the brain interprets as color.

It is this interplay of light, pigment, and vision that causes color to occur. Leaves look green because the pigment chlorophyll reflects green light. Leaves change color in the fall because they undergo a chemical change—the chlorophyll decomposes, exposing other pigments in the leaves that reflect other wavelengths of light. But if you were color blind, leaves might not look green at all, whether in spring or fall. And if there wasn't anyone there to *see* the leaves, the leaves wouldn't *appear* any color whatsoever. Ultimately, color, like sound, scent and pain, occurs in our minds.

Light is not everything that goes into the making of color, but it is certainly the *essence* of color. Without light, nothing has color. In darkness there is no color, because for there to be color there must be *light*. Imagine yourself in a huge room lit only by a single candle. You are looking around in the dimness. As your eyes travel away from the flame and into the shadows, colors become less distinct, then become degrees of gray, then completely disappear into blackness. Color is created by light, or contained in light.

The Color Spectrum

Light, radiant energy, travels in waves, like certain other forms of energy (radio waves, for instance). Light is made up of waves of different lengths. When light is separated by wavelength, or refracted, the result is a band of color, the **color spectrum,** or visible spectrum, which looks like a rainbow. White light contains the colors of the rainbow. Rainbows are the result of the dispersion of sunlight by water droplets in the sky. Prisms split light, too, displaying the color spectrum: red, orange, yellow, green, blue, and violet. Separating all the wavelengths of light makes the spectral band. Blending them all makes white light.

An object that looks blue is reflecting only the blue frequency of light. It absorbs all the other wavelengths and reflects only blue,

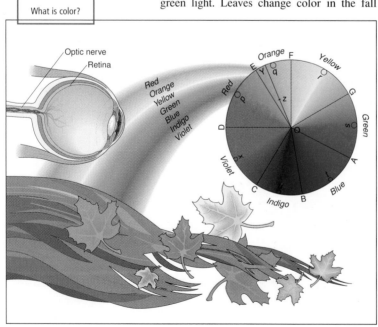

What is color?

Optic nerve
Retina

Red
Orange
Yellow
Green
Blue
Indigo
Violet

Orange
Yellow
Red
Green
Violet
Indigo
Blue

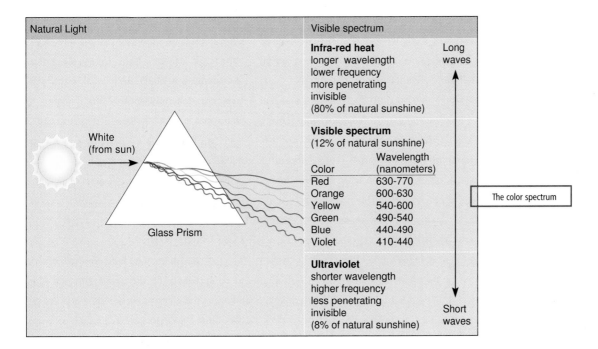

Natural Light		Visible spectrum	
		Infra-red heat longer wavelength lower frequency more penetrating invisible (80% of natural sunshine)	Long waves
		Visible spectrum (12% of natural sunshine)	
		Color	Wavelength (nanometers)
		Red	630-770
		Orange	600-630
		Yellow	540-600
		Green	490-540
		Blue	440-490
		Violet	410-440
		Ultraviolet shorter wavelength higher frequency less penetrating invisible (8% of natural sunshine)	Short waves

White (from sun)

Glass Prism

The color spectrum

which enters the eye. A red object absorbs all wavelengths but red—it reflects red and that is what the eye perceives. Black is the absorption of all light waves; white is the reflection of all light waves.

The human eye is only capable of perceiving certain wavelengths: the visible spectrum. You might say there is more "color" in the world than we can see!

Color Wheels

The order of the spectral colors is also the order of the colors on color wheels. The **color wheel** is a man-made invention, the purpose of which is to express the natural laws of color. There are many different versions of color wheels, each designed to emphasize one aspect or another of color theory. The great physicist Sir Isaac Newton was the first to explain prismatic effects and to describe the color spectrum (in the mid-1660s), and the first to position the spectral colors on a wheel. Many different color wheels have since been pro-

posed. In about 1731, J.C. Le Blon originated the theory of primary and secondary pigments. Color wheels use by hair-colorists display pigment colors, rather than spectral colors.

Optical Effects

We say that some colors are "warm" and others "cool." Optically, warm colors appear closer and cool colors seem more distant. Brighter colors (more toward orange or yellow) look harder; muted colors (more neutral or ash) look softer. Dark colors look more dense, light colors look airy. Colors interact to fool our eyes; a color standing alone looks different when it is placed beside another color.

Color Has Psychological Meaning

Color has a *psychological* side. Color, like fragrances and music, affects people emotionally. Color sends signals, even in nature, birds with the brightest plummage get the most attention! Colors evoke emotional responses: Bright colors are used in fast food

Color, like fragrances and music, affects people emotionally.

places to hurry you up, blues in hospital rooms to calm you down, white to convey cleanliness, not to mention the "green-eyed monster," "feeling blue," "in the pink," "seeing red," and so on. Colors have social and cultural meanings—white at a wedding, black for a funeral, pink for girls, and blue for boys. Haircolor also has some social meaning, which varies by region and era. What do we say about blonds? About redheads? About brassy hair in the rural south? Part of the reason why people want their hair a certain color is for what it says about them socially, which may be different in Beverly Hills, California, and Midland, Michigan, and different in 1950, 1975, and the year 2000.

The Importance of Lighting in the Salon

Have you ever been in a place, like in the cosmetics department of a retail store, selecting a shade of foundation, where you felt like you just couldn't see color clearly? Perhaps you really *couldn't* see it, not fully. You needed more light, or a different kind of light, to see its true color and when you got the foundation home, it looked different! More light had to strike it before you could see its full, true coloring.

Color comes from light; color is part of light. There can only be color when there is light. That is why it is so important to have good lighting in the salon for haircoloring. Otherwise, you literally can't see what you are doing. You need to be able to see the client's natural haircolor accurately, you need to be able to appreciate the coloring of her skin and eyes, and you want her to be able to accurately inspect the finished result!

Indirect natural daylight, or its artificial equivalent, shows the truest color. Dark walls absorb and decrease light; light walls reflect and increase light. Walls painted warm neutrals are generally most complimentary to skin—soft pink or golden undertones cast a healthy light on skin. Direct or bright light makes colors look more yellow or orange; diffused or dim light makes colors look more brown or gray.

LEVEL AND TONE

The first task in learning haircoloring theory is to comprehend the difference between *level* and *tone*. Level and tone are the words for the two most important characteristics of color. All haircolors, natural or artificial, have these two attributes.

Level

Level simply refers to the lightness or depth (darkness) of a haircolor, be it natural or artificial. Words such as *light, medium, dark, palest, darkest,* and *very light* tell you about a color's level. Level is, very simply, how light or how dark a haircolor is.

Numbers are used to indicate the level of colors. There are two main variations on the **Universal,** or **International, Level System:**

10. Very Light Blond	10. Lightest Blond
9. Light Blond	9. Very Light Blond
8. Medium Blond	8. Light Blond
7. Dark Blond	7. Medium Blond
6. Light Brown	6. Dark Blond
5. Medium Brown	5. Light Brown
4. Dark Brown	4. Medium Brown
3. Very Dark Brown	3. Dark Brown
2. Brown Black	2. Darkest Brown
1. Black	1. Black

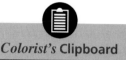

Colorist's Clipboard

What is color?

• *Color comes from light.*

• *Pigments alter light by absorbing some of the light and reflecting the rest. Reflected light enters the eye, and is what we interpret as color.*

• *For instance, carotenoids are pigments that make plants look yellow, orange, or red. Orange light bounces off a carrot, its pigments absorb everything but the orange light waves. The color of the carrot is due to the available light, the pigments in the carrot that make it reflect certain light rays, and the ability of your eyes to see the color orange.*

Manufacturers' level systems vary somewhat from one another. Some products have ten levels, some 11, some 12. A light brown may look darker in one system and lighter in another. It may be called a 6 level by one company and a 5 level by others.

Regardless of these variations, the lowest number (1 or 0) will be the darkest color in any given system. The highest number will represent the lightest color.

Levels are precise degrees of lightness or depth, standardized across the manufacturer's tonal groups. All colors of the same level will have the same degree of lightness or depth, whether natural (neutral), ash, gold, red, or any other tone.

To illustrate this, visualize a tall building, black at the basement and white at the penthouse, evenly graduating from dark to light, each story a grade lighter than the one beneath it. That's the International Level System, with numbers identifying those grades of dark to light. If you wash this image with a hue, such as gold, then you have a **tonal series.**

Look at, or imagine in your mind's eye, a black-and-white photograph. You are seeing only *levels* of color, not *tones* (although you may know or be able to guess what the tones are).

Tone

Tone refers to the *hue* of a haircolor, be it natural or artificial. The main tones, or hues, of haircoloring are natural (neutral), ash, gold, and red.

Manufacturers usually indicate the tones of their colors with letters: "A" for ash, "N" for natural (neutral), and so on. Numbers may also be used to designate tone; for instance, if ".1" means ash, then a 6 level ash would be "6.1."

Any color—haircolor or not—can be described, theoretically, in terms of level and tone. If a carpet is blue (tone) then how light or dark is it (level)? Is it a very dark blue, like navy? Is it nearly black, like ink? Is it somewhat deep, but not dark—medium—like royal blue? Or is it as pale as the pale blue sky? These are distinctions in level.

My husband's eyes are an 8 level blue. Just kidding! You can't plug a hue like blue into the International Level System because it isn't a haircolor (not usually). In theory you might, but not in reality. The level system pertains specifically and only to haircoloring.

If you are having trouble distinguishing between level and tone, give it time. It will come to you.

One caveat: if you take a painting class, or consult an art glossary, level and tone will be

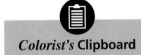

Colorist's **Clipboard**

Characteristics of color:

- *Level means how light or dark*

- *Tone means hue*

- *Intensity refers to the purity or strength of a tone*

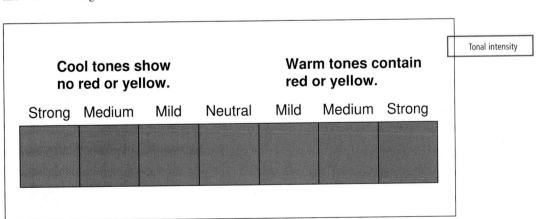

Tonal intensity

Cool tones show no red or yellow.   **Warm tones contain red or yellow.**

Strong	Medium	Mild	Neutral	Mild	Medium	Strong

defined differently. The painter's use of the words *tone, tint, shade*, and so forth, are not the same as the haircolorist's—each has different vernaculars.

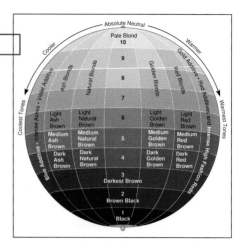

Munsell color sphere

Tonal Intensity

Intensity refers to the strength of a tone. Red-browns (auburns) are warm but not as intense as true reds. Even hotter than the true reds are the high-fashion reds and red additives. Auburns are warm, true reds are warmer (more intense), high-fashion reds and red additives are warmest (the most intense).

On the cool end of the spectrum, natural series colors are slightly cool, ash series colors are strongly cool, and "drabbers" are intensely ash. (Cool, cooler, coolest.)

The more intense the series, the less appropriate it is for gray hair. Intense colors (hot reds and the drabbest ashes) are designed to be used on pigmented hair. The purest, most intense colors are called concentrates, jewel tones, mixers, drabbers, intensifiers, fortifiers, and so on, and are usually too strong to be used alone.

The Munsell Color Sphere

American color theorist Albert Munsell explained level and tone this way: ". . . [L]et us substitute a geometric solid, like a sphere, and make use of geographical terms. The north pole is white. The south pole is black. The equator is a circuit of middle reds, yellows [and other hues] . . . above the equator [are] lighter values, and . . . below [are] darker values."[1]

Above is a haircolorist's adaptation of the **Munsell Sphere.**

At the equator are all the 5 level medium browns: medium natural brown, medium ash brown, medium golden brown, medium red brown. The Arctic Circle is palest blond—as light as hair gets—and Antarctica is as black as hair gets.

As you travel due north from the equator, hair gets lighter and lighter, within the same tonal series. Due south, hair gets darker and darker. Not all tones can be seen on the darkest hair. Warm-series colors can go only so deep, cool colors can be deeper. Most series trail off around a level 3 or 4.

Shade Systems versus Level Systems

Some color lines are not level systems at all, but shade systems. If a haircoloring product does not have precisely calibrated levels, with colors clearly identified by level and tone, it is a **shade system.** At the present time, the level system is much more common among professional products.

LUMINOSITY

The two most important characteristics of color are level and tone. Formulation is impossible without an understanding of level and tone.

There is another, related characteristic, which is helpful to acknowledge because it affects the way we perceive color, although it is not essential to the formulation process.

---

1 *A Color Notation, A. H. Munsell, 10th ed. (Baltimore, MD: Munsell Color Co., 1946), p. 18. Reprinted with the permission of Macbeth Div., Kollmorgen Instruments Corp. Munsell's Sphere is based on an earlier globe by the German painter Philipp Otto Runge (The Forms of Color, K. Gerstner, [MIT Press, 1986], pp. 12-14).*

Colorist's Clipboard

- *Warm colors reflect more light.*
- *Cool colors absorb more light.*

Luminosity, or **reflectivity,** refers to how much light a color reflects. Great light reflection lends brightness and *light*-ness. Warm colors reflect more light than cool colors. Therefore, warm colors appear shinier, brighter, and lighter than cool colors. Cool colors reflect less light than warm colors and, being less luminous, tend to look more matte or flat, and darker.

Do not attribute undue importance to this principle, but do tuck it away in the back of your mind. An awareness of light reflection may help you to identify natural levels with more accuracy, and to better understand the way different tones are perceived.

THE COLOR WHEEL (THE LAW OF COLOR)

Color wheel theory is not complicated. It can be presented in a complicated *fashion*, but it is not in itself complicated. If you have never really understood the color wheel, now is the time to understand it.

The **color wheel** is all about hue, or tone. Any hue you can imagine is somewhere on the color wheel. The color wheel shows how all the hues in the world relate to each other.

The color wheel assists in formulation by teaching what happens when different tones are mixed. The color wheel concept of warm

Sir Isaac Newton:

"But it's further to be noted that the most luminous of the prismatic colours are the yellow and orange. These affect the senses more strongly than all the rest together..."

—*from* Optics, *originally published in 1704* (Chicago, IL: Great Books, Encyclopaedia Brittanica, *1952*), *p. 418.*

Color wheel

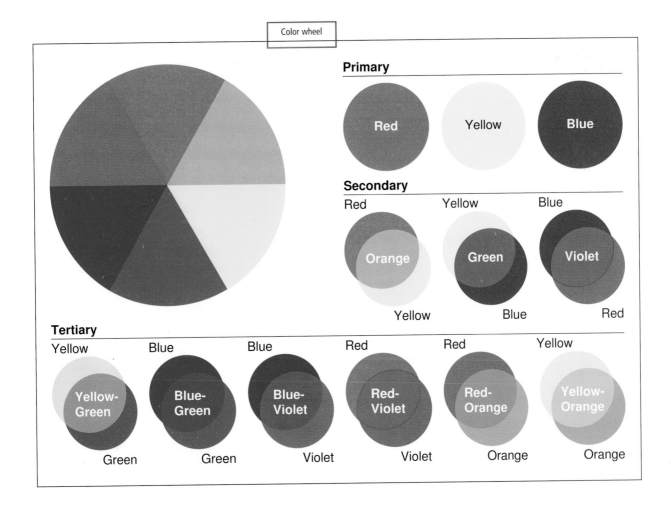

Primary

Red   Yellow   Blue

Secondary

Red   Yellow   Blue
Orange   Green   Violet
Yellow   Blue   Red

Tertiary

Yellow   Blue   Blue   Red   Red   Yellow
Yellow-Green   Blue-Green   Blue-Violet   Red-Violet   Red-Orange   Yellow-Orange
Green   Green   Violet   Violet   Orange   Orange

Draw Your Own Color Wheel

Primaries:

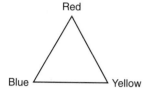

Secondaries:

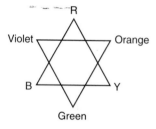

Tertiaries:

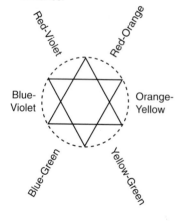

and cool colors helps the stylist communicate with clients and select appropriate tones for them, and also allows us to **neutralize,** or **contrast-out,** unwanted tones in the hair.

Primary Colors

A lesson on the color wheel must always start with the primary colors, because that's where all color begins. The word *primary* means "first." The **primary colors** are the first colors, the pigments from which all others are derived.

The primary pigments are *red, yellow,* and *blue.* These colors cannot be broken down into other colors. They are the elemental pigments. They are combined to create all other colors. For example: red cannot be broken down into other colors, but orange can be broken down—into red and yellow. Red and yellow are combined to create orange.

To draw your own color wheel, first make a triangle with three equal sides. Label each of its points with the name of a primary color.

If you have trouble recalling the primaries, then *Read Your Book!* *R*ed, *Y*ellow, *B*lue—get it? Now you will never forget them.

Of the primaries, yellow is the lightest and blue is the darkest. So, dark tints contain more blue pigment, and light tints contain more yellow pigment. Tints of a medium depth contain the most red pigment.

Secondary Colors

The secondary colors are the three pigments which are immediately derived from the primaries. The combination of two primary pigments, in equal parts, produces a **secondary color.**

There are three possible combinations of primary colors, each resulting in one of the secondary colors.

- *red* + *yellow* = **orange**
- *yellow* + *blue* = **green**
- *blue* + *red* = **violet**

The secondary colors are orange, green, and violet (or, you may prefer the word *purple*). To add the secondaries to your drawing of the color wheel, make another triangle, inverted and overlapping on the first triangle. Label each of its points with the name of a secondary color.[2]

There are many ways to demonstrate the principle of secondary colors. You have undoubtedly seen this principle in action—in your kitchen, in an art class, even on TV ("yellow and blue make green!" the announcer says, sealing the storage bag).

To make orange frosting for your Halloween cookies, what two food colors do you mix? Red and yellow, of course. And if a pink Easter egg falls into the blue dye—oops!— what do you get? Blue and pink (the lightest form of red) make violet (purple).

Watercolors are commonly used to demonstrate secondary colors. A child's palette is all you need. Just mix the primaries to get the secondaries.

Colored transparencies can also be used to demonstrate secondary colors. Transparencies in all of the primary colors can be found in art and office supply stores. Hold one up to a light source (like a window) and lay another over a big corner of it. The yellow transparency laid over the red makes orange, the blue over the red makes violet, and so on.

---

2 This version of the color wheel is most like the six-pointed star invented by Charles Blanc in 1873. Faber Birren presents a good history of color circles in *Principles of Color* (West Chester, PA: Schiffer, 1987).

Tertiary Colors

The primary pigments are red, yellow, and blue. The secondary pigments are orange, green, and violet. Now what about all the other colors? Teal (blue-green), plum (reddish-purple), chartreuse (yellowish-green)—how are these colors classified?

Blue-green, red-purple, and yellow-green are tertiary colors. Tertiary means "third"—the third phase of color. Tertiary colors are formed by mixing one primary and one of the secondaries next to it (on the color wheel), in equal parts. For example, red mixed with violet makes plum (red-violet). There are six tertiary pigments.

- *red-violet*
- *red-orange*
- *yellow-orange*
- *yellow-green*
- *blue-green*
- *blue-violet*

Cool versus Warm Colors

The color wheel can be divided into two hemispheres: warm colors on the right, and cool colors on the left.

Warm colors, which have the tone of something that imparts heat, range from yellow to red.

Cool colors are also called **ash,** meaning "what the fire leaves behind"—or the absence of warmth. Ash, or cool, colors range from green to violet.

At either "pole" of the color wheel, where the hemispheres meet, there is some overlap of cool and warm. A yellow tertiary can be greenish, and therefore cool. Yellows, or golds, sometimes tilt toward cool.

A red tertiary can be purplish, and therefore cool. Red-violets are *cool* reds. True reds, red-oranges, and red-golds are *warm* reds.

Knowledge of cool and warm tones is applied when selecting the appropriate haircoloring tone for a client. Some clients like, and look best in, warm tones; some like, and look best in, cool tones.

Contrasting Colors, or Complements

Complements are opposites on the color wheel. Colors which are opposite one another on the color wheel contrast-out each other, producing a neutral tone when combined.

Examples of **complementary pairs,** also known as **contrasting colors,** are yellow and violet, and red and green. Yellow contrasts-out violet, and vice-versa. Red and green contrast-out each other.

Notice that *one of the complements is always cool, and the other warm. Cool and warm contrast-out each other.* Ash eliminates warmth, and vice-versa.

Knowledge of contrasting colors is important in corrective haircoloring. The principle of complementary colors is used to neutralize unwanted tones in the hair. Which would be the most effective color to neutralize excessive gold (yellow) in the hair? Violet, of course. Which would best eliminate excessive orange? Blue neutralizes orange best. This is called **"browning-out," "balancing,"** or **"overtoning"** an unwanted tone.

Ash formulas are used in lightening to eliminate the natural red and gold that lightening exposes; ash contrasts-out excessive, unwanted warmth to net a more neutral result.

And, knowing that yellow and blue make green, the colorist won't put a bluish toner on hair prelightened to yellow!

Cool and Warm Colors

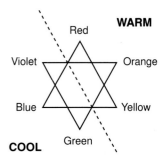

Complementary Colors

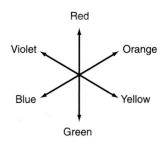

The Color Wheel (The Law of Color)

- *Primaries: red, yellow, and blue*

- *Secondaries: orange, green, and violet*

- *Tertiaries: red-violet, red-orange, yellow-orange, yellow-green, blue-green, and blue-violet*

- *Complementary pairs: colors opposite one another on the color wheel (examples are: yellow and violet, orange and blue, and red and green). Complements create a neutral tone when mixed.*

The word *complements* is not the same as *compliments*. The word *complementary* means "mutually supplying each other's lack."[3] One of a pair of complements will always be a secondary color and the other its "missing primary." When two complements are combined, all three primaries are present. That is why complements produce neutral tones. When all three primaries are mixed, a neutral tone is achieved. (Orange, made of red and yellow, is eliminated

by blue, its missing primary. Green, made of blue and yellow, is eliminated by red, the missing primary.)

CONCLUSION

The color wheel is simple. Remember the primaries. Knowing these, you can name the secondaries. Visualize these colors arranged on a circle. Half the circle is cool; half is warm. Colors opposite one another neutralize each other. Cool contrasts-out warm, and vice-versa. That's all you need to know.

---

3 Webster's New Collegiate Dictionary *(Spring-field, MA: G. & C. Merriam Co., 1975), p. 230.*

Violet vs. Purple

If we were discussing the color spectrum, we would use the word violet, and only the word violet, when speaking of that particular wavelength of light which gives us the color we perceive as red-blue. But we are not talking about the physics of light here; we are simply talking about color. Haircolorists are mainly concerned with color as it is perceived visually, not with frequencies of light. We deal in pigment and are concerned with the law of color as it pertains to pigment.

The spectral colors are not quite the same as pigment colors. The primary colors of light are different from the primaries of pigment. Color wheels pertaining to light are different from wheels pertaining to pigment. Color words have somewhat different meanings to physicists and artists or haircolorists.

In terms of pigment colors, either violet or purple is an acceptable label for the secondary color that results from the combination of red and blue. Although most stylists prefer the word violet, both violet and purple accurately describe the range of colors that is midway between red and blue on the color wheel. The two words broadly mean the same thing. The fact that we

have two words for one of the secondary colors is simply a peculiarity of the English language.

So it is not more accurate, technically, to say violet, rather than purple, when referring to the secondary color you get when you mix red and blue pigments.

However, violet and purple really are usually considered to be distinct tonally, though not everyone makes the same distinctions. Depending on the dictionary you consult or whom you ask, violet and purple may either be used interchangeably, or may be considered different, in one or both of the following two ways:

1. Violet has gray in it whereas purple is more pure. Violet is muted, less intense, less saturated, and softer (and usually lighter). Because it is "grayed down," violet is more suitable as a base color for haircoloring. Purple is clearer, more jewel-like, more brilliant, more concentrated, more intense, and stronger (and usually deeper).

2. Violet has more blue in it than purple does; purple has more red in it than violet does. Violet is more bluish (it is a reddish-blue), whereas purple is more reddish (it is a bluish-red).

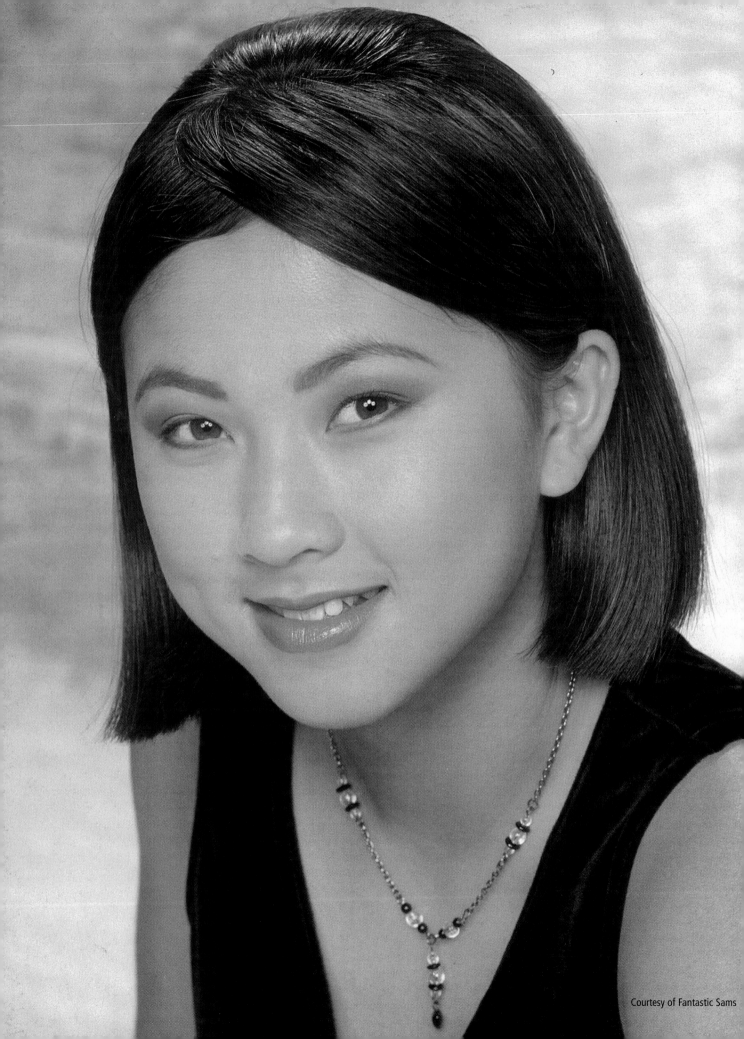

Courtesy of Fantastic Sams

hair structure and natural pigment

An understanding of the basic structure of hair is essential to understanding the haircoloring process; to know about haircoloring, you have to know about hair. This chapter is devoted to the general anatomy of hair, the nature of melanin, and the characteristics of hair that affect the haircoloring process.

BASIC HAIR STRUCTURE

Below the surface of the skin is the **hair root;** above it is the **hair shaft.**

The hair root is housed in a sheath, a pocket in the skin, called a **follicle.** At the bottom of the follicle, buried deep in the skin, is the **hair bulb.** The cells that become a strand of hair are produced in the hair bulb, the living part of hair, from which the hair grows. At the base of the bulb, nourishing it, is the **papilla,** a tiny mound of tissue laced with capillaries.

The hair shaft is comprised primarily of cross-linked, fibrous proteins called **keratin.** Keratin accounts for 90 to 95 percent of hair weight.

Structures in the hair bulb called **melanocytes** make **melanin,** or natural pigment, that gives the strand color. On average, 2 to 3 percent of the total weight of hair consists of melanin.

How is hair formed? The papilla supplies **amino acids** to the hair bulb; the hair bulb produces keratinous cells; melanocytes infuse melanin into these protein-based cells; then, finally, the cells dry out and harden to form the hair strand (called **keratinization**) which emerges from the follicle.

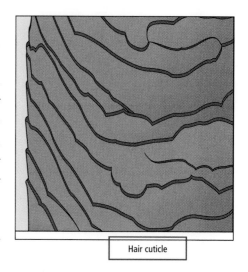

Hair cuticle

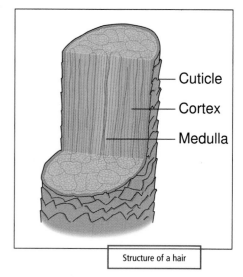

— Cuticle
— Cortex
— Medulla

Structure of a hair

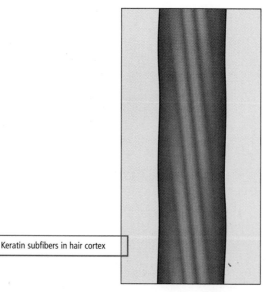

Keratin subfibers in hair cortex

A strand of hair has three principal layers: cuticle, cortex, and medulla.

The **cuticle** is the protective outer layer of the hair shaft. It is made of tough, resistant, high-sulfur keratin. The multiple, overlapping **cuticle scales** are often compared to the shingles of a roof, or a stack of paper cups nesting in one another. Hair averages seven to ten cuticle layers at midshaft. The cuticle is usually colorless, containing no melanin.

The **cortex** is the second and thickest layer of the hair strand. Nearly all the melanin of

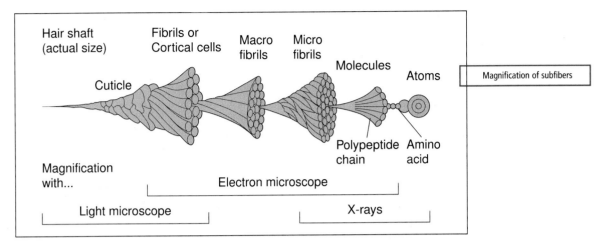

Hair shaft (actual size)

Fibrils or Cortical cells

Macro fibrils

Micro fibrils

Cuticle

Molecules

Atoms

Polypeptide chain

Amino acid

Magnification of subfibers

Magnification with...

Electron microscope

Light microscope

X-rays

hair resides in the **cortical layer.** The cortex consists of complex, ropelike keratin **fibrils,** surrounded by a **matrix** of protein, and cross-linked by **disulfide (cystine) bonds.** The cortex is the source of hair's great elastic strength.

The innermost layer is the **medulla,** which is considered nonessential. It may be intermittent, leaving off and starting up again, or, in fine hair, entirely absent.

MELANIN

Melanin is the pigment that gives hair its natural color. Melanin gives color to skin, too. How light or dark hair is naturally, and its characteristic natural tone, depends on how much and what kind of melanin it contains, and how that melanin is arranged in the hair.

The great majority of melanin is located in the cortical layer of the hair shaft, but the

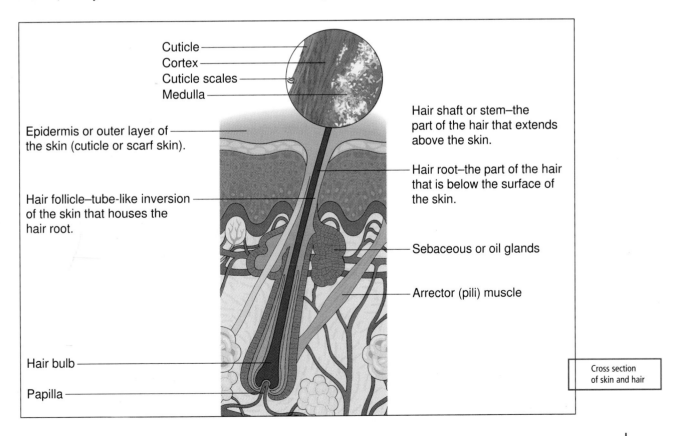

Cuticle
Cortex
Cuticle scales
Medulla

Epidermis or outer layer of the skin (cuticle or scarf skin).

Hair shaft or stem—the part of the hair that extends above the skin.

Hair root—the part of the hair that is below the surface of the skin.

Hair follicle—tube-like inversion of the skin that houses the hair root.

Sebaceous or oil glands

Arrector (pili) muscle

Hair bulb

Papilla

Cross section of skin and hair

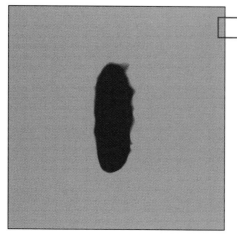

A melanin molecule

There are two main types of melanin.

- **Eumelanins (eumelanosomes) are the darker pigments, ranging from black to brown.**
- **Pheomelanins (pheomelanosomes) are lighter, ranging from red-brown to red-yellow to yellow.**

All hair, no matter what color it is (with the exception of pure white hair, which is unpigmented), may contain both eumelanin and pheomelanin in varying amounts and degrees of dispersion or aggregation. Very black Asian or African hair is heavily pigmented but may contain only eumelanin.

The color of a strand of hair depends on: how much melanin it contains, the proportion of eumelanin to pheomelanin, and the pattern of distribution of the melanin—whether it is more granular (clustered together) or more diffused (more scattered about in the hair shaft).

medulla contains melanin, too, and melanin is occasionally, though infrequently, found in the cuticle (and then usually only in the blackest hair). Melanin is made by cells in the hair bulb called melanocytes. During keratinization, melanin is infused into the protein that becomes the hair strand, in the form of pigment granules, or **melanosomes.**

Melanin is pigment and protein, or pigment *in* protein, called **melanoprotein.** Melanosomes are protein-coated granules of pigment.

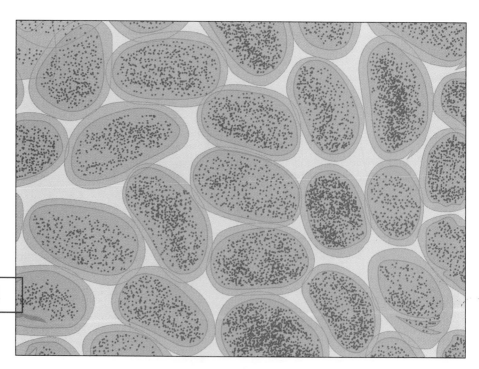

Cross section of hairs showing natural pigments in auburn hair

The darkest hair has the most melanin, a preponderance of eumelanin, and the largest melanin granules. Blond hair has less melanin than dark hair, less eumelanin than pheomelanin, and smaller, more-diffused melanin granules. Gray strands have very little melanin—next to none—and the purest white hair (such as albino hair) has no melanin at all. Melanin may account for as much as 4 percent of the total weight of very black hair, whereas dark blond hair may contain only .2 or .5 percent melanin.

A third type of pigment, tricochromes, is sometimes mentioned in haircoloring literature. It does not occur in all hair and is far less prevalent than eumelanin or pheomelanin. The **tricochromes** are yellow-red pigments found especially in carrot-red hair; they are related to, but not the same as, pheomelanin.

THE LIGHTENING OF MELANIN

From the colorist's point of view, the most important thing to know about melanin is what happens to it in the presence of haircoloring. The color result depends as much on the natural pigmentation of the hair as it does on the artificial pigment used; the same ash brown formula may look orange-y on one natural base, drab on another, and neutral on a third. Recognizing what depth the hair is to start with and how it will change tonally when lightened allows you to anticipate the final result.

Through the years, manufacturers have devised different ways of getting this across to hairdressers. Depending on your product orientation, and on how long you've been in the business, you probably subscribe to certain terminology and explanations related to the lightening of hair. Brand R talks about it in a certain way, Brand C offers another explanation, Brands L and M have their way of teaching.

But the point of any theory of lightening is to drive home the idea that the color result depends on more than what you put in the bowl—it also depends on the color contribution of the hair. Natural color contribution depends on: 1) the original virgin color, and 2) how much you lighten it.

The natural base level, and the lightening capability of your formula, determine the color contribution of the hair.

The color contribution of the hair, and the artificial pigment used, determine the color result.

Natural color + the lightening capability of the formula = the color contribution of the hair (AND) The color contribution of the hair + the artificial pigment = the color result.

"Color contribution of the hair" is expressed different ways by the various haircoloring companies: undertones, underlying pigment, natural underlying pigmentation, pigment bases, residual pigment contribution, natural contribution of the hair, lightened natural pigment, and remaining natural color.

Any one of these terms can be substituted in that last equation:

lightened natural pigment + artificial pigment = the color result (OR) remaining natural color + artificial pigment = the color result.

With no-lift demi-permanents and semi-permanents, lightening is not a consideration, but the result will still vary according to the

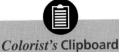

Colorist's Clipboard

Melanin:

• There are two main types of melanin: eumelanin (black to brown), and pheomelanin (red to yellow).

• Natural haircolor depends on: how much melanin the hair contains, the proportion of eumelanin to pheomelanin, and whether the melanin is more diffused (scattered) or granular (clustered).

base level, or natural pigment, of the hair (natural color + artificial pigment = the color result).

Seven Stages of Lightening

This concept concerns the color changes that occur when hair is exposed to a product capable of lightening. It is primarily a teaching tool, and not necessarily a literal explanation of what occurs as hair is lightened.

One of the most essential lessons in haircoloring is that the final result depends as much on the natural contribution of the hair as it does on the artificial dyes, and the seven stages of lightening is a way of expressing that. It is one of the theories of lightening most familiar to hairstylists.

The **seven stages of lightening** are the colors that hair attains as it is lightened with either permanent haircoloring or bleach. Theoretically, if hair bleaching could be viewed in slow motion, these are the tonal stages that would be seen during the progression from dark to light. The seven stages of lightening are:

1. BLACK
2. BROWN
3. RED
4. RED-GOLD
5. GOLD
6. YELLOW
7. PALE YELLOW

When hair is exposed to a lightening agent, its black and brown pigments are first to begin to break down or oxidize (the eumelanin lightens first). Then the red and gold pigments gradually oxidize (pheomelanin is more resistant to lightening). The yellow and pale yellow stages are simply lighter and lighter versions of gold.

When natural pigment oxidizes in the sun, it lightens similarly. Exposed to sun, brown hair becomes reddish and blond hair becomes golden. The ashy eumelanin begins oxidizing first, leaving warmth prominent in the hair.

Notice that five of the seven stages have to do with red and gold. This is due to the relative tenacity of these colors in the hair. It simply takes longer to eliminate red, and longer still to eliminate gold. Gold is the most difficult pigment color to eliminate.

We say that *lightening creates warmth*. The natural warmth of the hair is exposed when hair is lightened. That's why ash formulas are so often used to lift: in order to contrast-out the natural warmth that lightening creates.

The lightest of the seven stages, pale yellow, is often likened to the inside of a lemon, or the inside of a banana peel. (The next-to-lightest stage, yellow, is like the outside of a lemon.) Pale yellow is the lightest hair can become without being destroyed. Pale yellow hair can be *toned,* if desired, to appear whitish (or any other tone).

A haircoloring result is the combined effect of the natural pigment and the haircoloring formula.

Lightened natural pigment + artificial pigment = the color result.

The result achieved depends equally on the artificial pigment used and whatever natural pigment remains in the hair. For this reason, the stage of lightening might be considered fully 50 percent of the color result.

What Happens When Hair Is Lightened?
Realistically, lightening does not occur in precise stages, but as a continuum. When hair is exposed to hydrogen peroxide (or other bleaching agents), the granules of melanin are progressively dissolved. Depending on the strength of the lightener and the processing

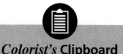

Colorist's **Clipboard**

What happens when melanin is lightened?

• As hair is lightened, natural underlying warmth is exposed; lightening creates warmth.

• Lightened natural pigment + artificial pigment = the color result.

time, part or all of the melanin may be dissolved. This dissolved pigment is then gradually dispersed and the hair becomes lighter and lighter in appearance.

Hydrogen peroxide (H_2O_2) supplies the oxygen to kinetically break up melanin. H_2O_2 has an affinity for melanin; it efficiently forces the melanin apart. Oxygen molecules released from the hydrogen peroxide assault the color granules with enough force to knock them apart.

When hair is lightened, eumelanin is affected first. Partially oxidized eumelanin (**oxymelanin**) probably looks like pheomelanin—reddish or golden in appearance. Very soon after lightening is under way, orange-y tones become apparent in the hair. As eumelanin is eliminated, pheomelanin in the hair becomes more apparent.

While largely lacking in pigmentation, gray hair also displays warmth when lightened. Even the most silvery hair is yellowed by bleaching.

DOMINANT UNDERLYING COLOR

There are numerous terms for underlying color: undertones, pigment bases, residual pigment contribution, remaining natural color, natural contribution of the hair, natural underlying pigmentation, and so forth. These terms all mean essentially the same thing—all refer to the color tone dominant in natural haircolor. The dominant, natural underlying color must always be considered when formulating, because it always affects the color result, so every haircoloring company has come up with their own way of talking about it. Whichever phrase you are most comfortable with is fine. In this book, the term most often used is "dominant underlying color."

Dominant underlying color is the dominant natural color tone which underlies a given level of haircolor. Each level of natural haircolor can be said to have one identifiable, dominant tone. It is that specific tone that makes that haircolor what it is, in terms of its depth or lightness.

Remember: Naturally pigmented hair contains a mixture of eumelanin and pheomelanin, in varying amounts, proportions, and patterns of distribution, to make the hair dark, medium, or light. You might think of the natural pigmentation of hair in terms of four basic colors: black, brown, red, and gold. It is the ratio of these colors to each other that makes hair dark, light, or somewhere in-between. Any given level of natural haircolor can be said to have more of one specific pigment color than any other.

For example, 5 level medium-brown hair can be said to contain more *red* than anything else. When medium-brown hair is lightened in the sun, it becomes reddish. When medium-brown hair is blonded with permanent haircoloring, lots of ash must be used to contrast-out its strong natural warmth. A client with a natural level of medium brown makes a good redhead, because she has lots of red naturally (it is easier to make her red and keep her red). The dominant underlying color of medium-brown hair is red.

The dominant underlying color of 6 level light-brown hair is *golden red,* or *dark orange.* Lightened by sunlight or perm chemicals, light-brown clients become orange-y (brassy).

7 level dark-blond hair has more gold than red; *reddish-gold,* or *light orange,* is predominant in dark-blond hair, and 8 level medium-blond hair has more *gold* than anything else. Natural blonds become golden in the sun.

This concept is closely related to, but not exactly the same as, the seven stages of lightening. It is a level system adaptation of the

Dr. Leszek J. Wolfram:
world-renowned cosmetic chemist:

"What happens to pigment when it is lightened by peroxide (or persulfates, which are much more aggressive) is a two-step process. First, the granules begin to dissolve—the pigment takes the form of a solution, not a granule—as though you had taken a powdered dye that you bought in a store and dissolved it in water. Although the melanin is dissolved (and you may finish up with total granule destruction) the hair is still colored at this point. Then, secondly, the dissolved melanin is further oxidized (broken down) to lighter colors . . .

"Seven stages of lightening is an arbitrary measure. You could say six stages, or eight, or ten. Lightening produces continuous color change."

Each level of natural haircolor can be said to have one identifiable, dominant tone, its dominant underlying color.

seven stages of lightening. Again, it is an invaluable teaching concept.

Every manufacturer of salon haircoloring will provide either a chart or a description of their level system's underlying colors, perhaps an implied description. (You may have to read between the lines to find it, perhaps in the information on color fillers, for instance.) Any good level system can be plugged into an undertone chart. Table 2-1 shows two typical charts.

These two charts are quite standard. The chart for your haircoloring product may vary, but it will be only slightly different. Manufacturers' level systems are all a little different, so one of the levels shown may be omitted, or the names for the various underlying hues may be slightly different, especially in the orange-to-gold stages. If there are additional very light blonds, they all have the same pale yellow undertone.

The major difference among undertone charts is what they have to say about the residual pigment of the darkest levels. Some companies describe the underlying color of the darkest levels in neutral terms (black or brown); some describe it as being blue and violet.

These charts and the concept of dominant underlying color are about *natural* pigment, not artificial pigment. Underlying color charts show the natural pigment color that is dominant within each natural base level. The study of natural pigment does lend some insight into the color composition of artificial dyes, but that is not of great concern here.

Two typical dominant underlying color charts

Natural Level	Dominant Underlying Color
Very Light Blond	Pale Yellow (Yellow-White)
Light Blond	Yellow
Medium Blond	Gold (Yellow-Orange)
Dark Blond	Reddish Gold (Light Orange)
Light Brown	Golden Red (Dark Orange or Red-Orange)
Medium Brown	Red
Dark Brown	Red-Brown
Very Dark Brown	Brown
Darkest Brown	Brown-Black
Black	Black

Natural Level	Dominant Underlying Color
Very Light Blond	Pale Yellow
Light Blond	Yellow
Medium Blond	Gold
Dark Blond	Light Orange
Light Brown	Dark Orange
Medium Brown	Red
Dark Brown	Red-Violet
Very Dark Brown	Violet
Darkest Brown	Blue-Violet
Black	Blue

TABLE 2-1

The Importance of the Concept of Dominant Underlying Color

Dominant underlying color and the seven stages of lightening are important for the same reason: *a haircoloring result is the combined effect of the artificial color and the remaining natural color.*

The result achieved depends equally on the artificial pigment you use and what natural pigment remains in the hair.

Artificial pigment
+ lightened natural pigment
= the color result.

To get the right color result, you have to get the right combination of artificial and remaining natural pigment. Dominant underlying color is therefore virtually 50 percent of the color result.

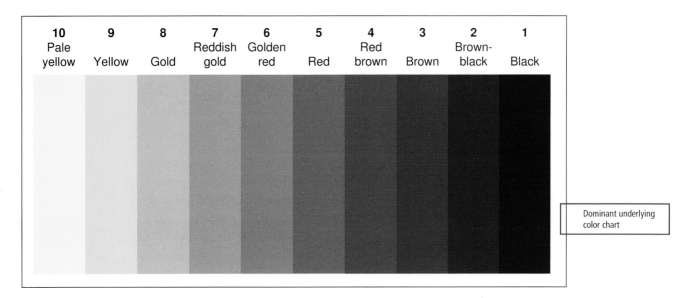

10 Pale yellow	9 Yellow	8 Gold	7 Reddish gold	6 Golden red	5 Red	4 Red brown	3 Brown	2 Brown-black	1 Black

Dominant underlying color chart

Look again at the charts in Table 2-1. If you are lightening from a natural level of dark brown to light brown, the dominant underlying tone remaining in the hair will be dark orange. If you do not want a warm result, then an ash formula is used to neutralize the natural orange color that will remain in the hair.

If dark-brown hair is to be lifted to blond, great warmth must be overcome. The hair must be lifted through the tenacious red and orange stages.

If you are trying to promote warmth in the hair, then natural underlying warmth is, of course, an asset. Artificial red-browns, reds, and golds will look better and hold better if there is natural warmth in the hair. The natural underlying warmth rounds out and supports the artificial warmth, enhancing the tone and longevity of the resulting color. (That is why it is easier to keep a client red who has natural brown hair than it is to keep red haircoloring in natural blond hair.)

Dominant Underlying Color and Double-Process Lightening

The concept of underlying color is crucial to **bleach-and-tone processes.** To successfully tone with the chosen tint or toner, the hair must be lightened to a prescribed stage of lightening (usually yellow or pale yellow). The appropriate natural undertone must be supplied or the toner will not have the desired effect.

Lighten too much, and the result will be unnaturally drab or off-color. Lighten too little, and the color result will be untoned-looking and overly yellowish.

Dominant Underlying Color and Color Fillers

The purpose of a **color filler** is to replace missing underlying pigment and compensate for overporosity. Fillers are always warm, because natural underlying pigment is warm. The color filler selected is generally slightly lighter than the dominant undertone of the level you intend to achieve. If the desired level is medium brown, for instance, dark orange is used to prepigment.

Compare the dominant underlying color chart with the filler recommendations in your manufacturer's literature. The two should be very close, either duplicates or about a level variant.

Dominant Underlying Color and Color Removal

The principle of dominant underlying color pertains to the lightening of artificial tint as much as it pertains to any lightening service.

Bleach, or a color remover, is used to lighten artificial tint. The hair progresses through warm stages similar to the lightening of natural pigment. When the hair is slightly lighter than the dominant underlying color of the target level, it is light enough to accept that level of tint. For instance, a client who has been previously tinted dark brown wishes to be light brown. The previous tint would be lifted to light orange, and then the client could be colored light brown. To lighten the hair *more* would make filling necessary. To lighten it *less* would cause warmth to bleed through.

Dominant Underlying Color and Gray Hair

Gray, or **white,** hair occurs when the hair bulb stops producing melanin. Gray hair is basically unpigmented: it contains little underlying pigment, or none at all.

The concept of dominant underlying color helps to explain the way gray hair accepts artificial coloring. Cool colors do not cover gray as well as warm colors, because they do not contain what gray hair lacks. Warm haircoloring replaces the missing warm undertones, in effect filling (prepigmenting) the hair.

THE EFFECT OF TEXTURE AND POROSITY

Manufacturers write formulation recommendations with average, normal hair in mind—that is, medium texture and normal porosity. For very coarse hair, very fine hair, resistant hair, or overporous hair, adjustments may be necessary.

Both the diameter of the hair strands (texture) and the condition of the cuticle (porosity) significantly affect color acceptance.

Texture and Its Effect on Haircoloring

Texture refers to the diameter of the individual hair strands. Is the hair fine, medium, or coarse? The greater the diameter of the hair shaft, the coarser the hair. The less the diameter, the finer the hair.

"Texture" also refers to the general feel of hair, which is a function of both diameter and condition. Sometimes the meaning of the word is further expanded to encompass **configuration:** straight, wavy, or curly. But for purposes of haircoloring, it is diameter that matters: is the hair fine, medium, or coarse?

Coarse hair has a thick cortex. Color chemicals must penetrate more mass and lift more natural pigment, so it takes longer to penetrate and lighten coarse hair. More processing time, a somewhat stronger developer, and an ashier formula (to eliminate greater natural underlying warmth) may be necessary when coloring very coarse hair.

The main difference between coarse hair and fine hair is the ratio of cuticle to the total weight of the hair strand. Coarse hair has proportionately more cortex and less cuticle. It has less surface area relative to its total weight, so it takes longer for chemicals to diffuse into it.

Fine hair has a thinner cortex, perhaps no medulla, and more surface area per its unit weight (a high proportion of cuticle). Therefore fine hair is penetrated more quickly. Less cortex means less melanin, so fine hair is also lightened more easily. Coloring is faster. Fine hair also fades faster, because it accepts less artificial pigment to start with (there is less room for dye molecules in the thinner hair shaft), and it has relatively more surface area for **fadage** to occur.

Ethnicity influences texture somewhat. Caucasian hair tends to be finer than other ethnic groups; African-American, Asian, and Native-American hair tend to be coarser. But the range of fine-to-coarse texture exists in every racial group, and each client must be evaluated individually.

We say fine hair is "baby fine" (or the less polite "frog fur"); coarse hair is "coarse as a horse's tail." Hair which is neither unusually fine nor unusually coarse is medium (average). Most people have **medium texture,** not fine and not coarse. More people perceive their hair to be finer or coarser than is really the case.

You will occasionally have a client with otherwise medium texture but a very fine hairline. A fine hairline lightens faster and has less underlying pigment to tone-out. It deepens more when depositing color. In applying color to this client, the fine hairline should be the last area to get color. Leave the hairline out until you are done applying to the rest of the hair, and strand-test if in doubt.

Porosity

Porosity is the ability of hair to absorb and retain moisture, determined by how raised or compact the cuticle layers are. Porosity is commonly referred to as the *condition* of the hair.[1]

Degrees of Porosity: Resistant, Normal, and Overporous

Depending on the condition of its cuticle layers, hair is classified as:

- *Resistant,*
- *Normal porosity, or*
- *Overporous.*

---

1 *This use of the word* porosity *has been disputed in the past.* Porous, *as the dictionary defines it, means "having pores"—and of course, hair does* not *have pores. Nonetheless, porosity has become accepted in common usage to mean "condition, or the ability of hair to absorb and retain moisture."*

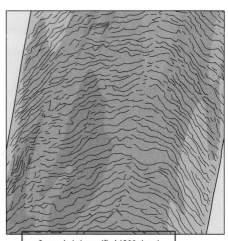

Coarse hair (magnified 1200 times)

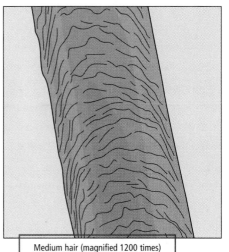

Medium hair (magnified 1200 times)

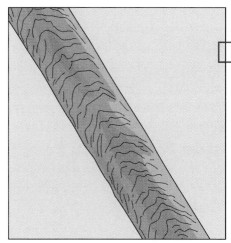

Fine hair (magnified 1200 times)

The words *resistant* and *tenacious* mean the same thing. A **tenacious,** or **resistant,** head of hair has a compact, unlifted cuticle which will resist absorption. The surface of the hair is slick, smooth, and shiny. Resistant hair is sometimes said to have "poor porosity."

Tenacity is seen and felt. A tight cuticle makes hair glossy, wiry, slick-looking, and slick to the touch. If you pick up a thin section and run your fingers down it, ends to scalp, you hardly feel an imbrication. We say it is "too healthy" (difficult to penetrate). Gray hair, Asian, Hispanic, and Native-American hair are all frequently tenacious.

A slightly raised cuticle (not compact, but not rough, either) indicates **normal porosity.** It is normal for hair to have a slightly raised cuticle because everything hair is exposed to creates porosity: sunshine, brushing, combing, shampooing, chlorine, and hair dryers and other thermal styling tools all "weather" hair, lifting and eroding cuticle scales.

A highly raised cuticle indicates **overporosity.** Overporous hair will appear ruffled and dull, without shine. It looks and feels rough. Pick up a thin section and run your fingers down it, ends to scalp, and it will backcomb in your fingers. Overporous hair is the opposite of resistant hair.

It is usually a combination of factors that results in overporosity. Color and perm chemicals have an immediate and obvious effect on porosity (any penetrating substance must expand the cuticle in order to work) and, of course, some chemicals are harsher than others. Sun and heat styling contribute—sometimes greatly—to cuticle damage. In addition, some hair is simply more vulnerable. If the hair is fragile to start with, then a permanent

wave, relaxer, or other **reforming service** will limit coloring options.

It is helpful to distinguish between **moderate overporosity** and **extreme overporosity.** *Moderate* means "medium"—not slight and not extreme. Professional **high-lift tint** usually makes hair moderately overporous. The combination of an excellent, salon-quality perm or relaxer and standard 20 volume color usually makes hair moderately overporous. Add a third factor—like neglect, excessive sun, or abusive heat styling—and now the hair is extremely overporous. A badly overprocessed perm will make hair extremely overporous.

The Effect of Porosity on Haircoloring
Resistant hair takes longer than average to soften and penetrate. This is known as "**underacceptance.**" Hair which is resistant should be allowed maximum timing. Very-low developer volumes (less than 15 to 20 volume) won't soften it sufficiently. Tenacious gray hair sometimes requires presoftening or prepigmentation.

Hair of *normal porosity* accepts and retains color normally. A slightly open cuticle allows color chemicals in normally and, once the coloring process is complete, closes enough to prevent dye molecules from escaping. Timing and formulation are normal for hair of normal porosity.

Overporous hair sponges up color—it drinks it—but it releases color quickly, too. It lets it in and lets it out. This is known as "**overacceptance.**" A highly raised cuticle is penetrated instantly (so timing is shorter) but it is not compact and intact enough to retain color molecules normally. Overporous hair tends to fade and may require filling. High volume developers are generally unnecessary and can

Overporous hair accepts dyes differently than hair of normal porosity.

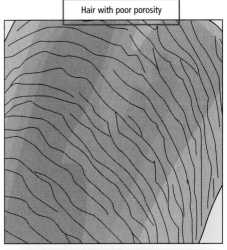

Hair with poor porosity

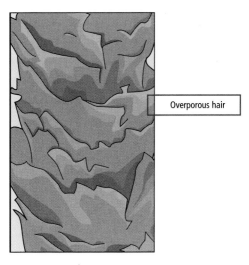

Overporous hair

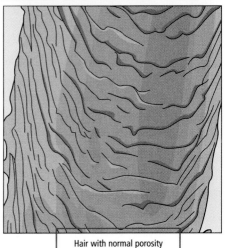

Hair with normal porosity

be quite detrimental on extremely overporous hair. If the color service is deposit-only, a low- or no-peroxide color is a gentle alternative (demi-permanent or semi-permanent products may be especially suitable).

Overporous hair accepts dyes differently than hair of normal porosity. The more overporous the hair, the more selective its acceptance of oxidation dyes. *With permanent haircoloring, overporous hair tends to reject warm artificial pigment (red and gold) and accept ash (cool or drab) pigment.* This is called **abused rejection.** Any ash pigment that happens to be in the color formula will develop readily in overporous hair. For this reason, formulas are adapted for overporosity by

increasing warmth. Because the hair will throw it off, you put more red or gold in the formula to start with. The greater the overporosity, the more extreme the inclination to be drab and dark, and the warmer the formula must be. Extremely overporous hair must be prepigmented in order to achieve an even and durable result.

When it comes to permanent haircoloring, damaged hair tends to go drab, and healthy hair tends to display warmth. With healthy hair, you fight (or make use of) warm undertones; with damaged hair you fight (or make use of) a tendency to go ash.

The direct dyes of semi-permanent haircoloring, though, are different. Damaged, overporous hair will pick up more of whatever direct dye is applied to it—more tone and more depth. On overporous hair, semi-permanent reds are redder, ashes are ashier, and dark colors are darker, whereas resistant hair absorbs much less color. This is true of temporary products, as well.

Keep this in mind about porosity: It lasts forever. Once the cuticle is lifted, there is no returning it to its virginal, compact state. Any porosity you create will remain forever, until the hair is cut off and gone.

Although normal porosity cannot be restored once lost, treatments designed to repair cuticle and cortical damage are of great value. The cuticle can be smoothed down and filled in (and should be, if the hair is overporous). This helps prevent further damage, makes the hair look better, and helps color take more evenly. But cuticle scales that are lifted can't be "nailed down," and scales that are broken off can't be pasted back on! Once hair is made overporous, it is overporous until it is cut off, and formulation or timing must always reflect that.

Multiporous Hair

When hair is overporous, it is usually only overporous on the ends, or on the ends and **midshaft.** The scalp area is almost always undamaged and normal, and frequently the midshaft is normal, as well. Ends are always the most porous area of the hair. This is where the term **multiporous** comes from, meaning "different porosities down the length of the hair." Almost without exception, a client with overporous hair will really be multiporous.

Permanent haircoloring on overporous ends tends to go darker and drabber. Auburn (red brown) haircoloring pulled through overporous ends without adjustment will be browner (less red) on the ends. Ash blond haircoloring pulled through overporous ends will go drab (muddy, flat, or off-tone). On extremely overporous ends, even neutral or slightly warm haircoloring will appear drab. Dark, drab ends make haircoloring look amateurish; professional color is *even* color. Generally speaking, if varying at all, commercial haircoloring should be lighter and brighter on the ends.

Excessively Damaged Hair

There is a degree of damage beyond even extreme overporosity. The cuticle can be so abraded—broken up and broken off—that the hair is just worn to tatters. The common term is "really fried" (not just "fried," but *really fried*"). This hair is more than extremely overporous; it is so utterly abused and direly overporous, so dry and weak, it is inelastic and breakable. Without proper treatment (and sometimes in spite of it) it will begin breaking off.

No matter where you live, chemical services gone awry can spell disaster, but the greatest extremes of overporosity are found in regions where the environment is adverse to healthy hair. Desert and sunny coastal areas are the most adverse—aridity, hard water, and salt water are damaging, and most abusive of all is sun. Sun converts cystine to cysteic acid as it lightens hair (like any oxidative process), degrading disulfide bonds and weakening the protein structure of hair. Sunscreens that are left in the hair do reduce sun damage and belong on your retail shelves. Neglect (abusive styling or lack of proper conditioning) compounds environmental damage. Some hair is simply more delicate, too—it cannot endure much chemical or environmental injury.

Hair of all degrees of overporosity can be colored (given proper product selection and formulation) with one exception. Hair that is so damaged that it is already breaking off is not hair which should be chemically treated. (It is a crass old joke, but it happens: "fried, dyed, and laid to the side.") If hairs break off when you squeeze the client's mane in your hand, don't try to color her—hair that is breaking off should be cut off, and the remaining hair properly treated, to moisturize and strengthen it, before coloring. This is better than having it break in the shampoo bowl.

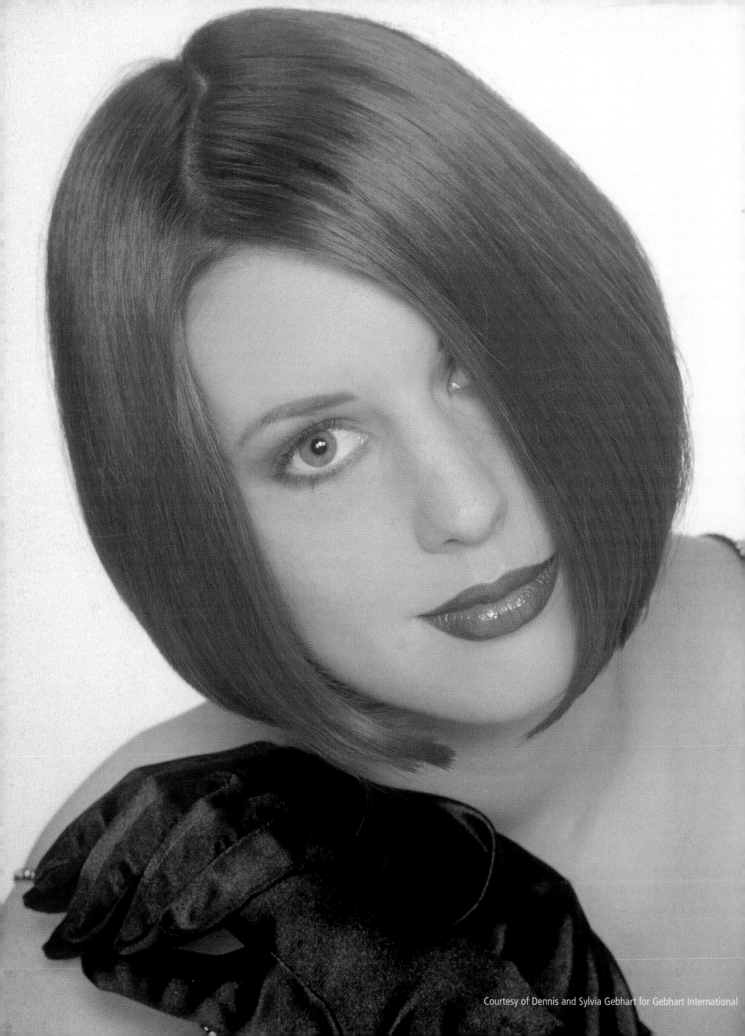

categories of haircoloring products

With advances in technology and the subsequent introduction of new and different haircoloring products, the lines between the conventional categories are not so sharply drawn as they once were. In some cases, the lines are downright blurry. Many products have attributes of more than one category and are hard to classify.

An understanding of the conventional haircoloring categories is as essential as ever, however. To match clients to products, to select the best product for a given client, the stylist must understand what's available, and the words *temporary, semi-permanent,* and *permanent* are the words we use in this industry to describe our haircoloring products—and now, *demi-permanent!* The addition of this fourth category, or subcategory, eliminates some previous ambiguities regarding semi-permanents.

Distinctions between the conventional categories still apply. But remember: Every product must be evaluated on its own merits, individually. It takes more than a single term to describe haircoloring products today. (And manufacturers are more than happy to tell you exactly what their products do!)

TEMPORARY HAIRCOLORING

Temporary haircoloring products are designed to last shampoo to shampoo. The mark of a temporary product is that it washes out, completely or almost completely, in a single shampoo. This category includes temporary rinses, most colored shampoos and conditioners, and most colored styling and finishing products (pigmented gels, mousses, pomades, and sprays). Touch-up crayons, once commonly used to conceal a gray regrowth between retouches, are still found in some drugstores. Forms of temporary color come and go (so to speak!), rising and falling in popularity: powders, glitters, gels, shellacs, lacquers, waxes, and paints.

In order to be truly temporary, a product must be **surface-acting.** Temporary products color the surface of the hair, superficially. They are formulated to *prohibit* penetration of the cuticle; high-weight dye molecules that cannot pass into the cortex are used. Temporary products do not affect natural pigment, either. In order to be temporary, obviously, a product cannot lighten natural pigment.

Temporary rinses and colored shampoos and moisturizers are generally water-based, water-soluble, acidic in pH, and are applied to the hair when it is damp and the cuticle is slightly expanded. The dye molecules of temporary products are much larger than the dyes of permanent haircoloring, and are generally larger than those of semi-permanent haircoloring, as well. Such big color molecules cannot pass into the cortex. They lodge between, and on, the cuticle scales and stick to the hair as it dries. The labels of temporary products may list acid dyes, basic dyes, and FD&C and D&C dyes.

Because the dye molecules of temporary haircoloring lay on top of the hair, and because they are such large molecules, temporary products, if overused, reduce natural shine and translucency. Hair with too much temporary color on it looks dull and unnatural.

Temporary products are porosity sensitive: the dye molecules settle in the hair where porosity permits. More porous hair traps more color; less color sticks to the slick, unbroken surface of resistant hair.

It is possible for a build-up of temporary haircoloring to occur. Temporary products are meant to be applied only as needed, not necessarily every time the hair is shampooed. (*All* haircoloring products are meant to be applied only as needed.) It is possible, therefore, to overuse these products and create a build-up. Furthermore, hair is usually heat-styled after application of a colored rinse or shampoo (blower and iron, or hood dryer), and any use of heat increases penetration and tends to fasten color molecules to the hair.

By definition, temporary haircoloring products should shampoo out. If considerable artificial color is still present after thorough shampooing, then there is a build-up in the hair which may affect other haircoloring services. For instance, a partly gray client has for years received brown rinses; now she wants blond permanent haircoloring. After thorough shampooing, her overporous ends still show a build-up of the temporary color. If her ends are deeper than the desired blond, she will have uneven color; her ends will remain darker than the rest of her hair. The permanent haircoloring will lift only her natural pigment. (Haircoloring does not lighten artificial pigment, as a rule.) To achieve an even result, it will be necessary to remove the dark residue on the ends of her hair prior to tinting her blond.

Whenever it is necessary to remove temporary color, it is a good idea to consult the manufacturer of the product to be removed. Different methods of removal are more or less effective with different products. Oil-based removers or clarifying treatments remove some temporary haircoloring (most clarifying shampoos can be used as treatments, too: lather, cover with a plastic cap, and process under a hood dryer for 15 minutes). Other temporary dyes may require decolorizing with a peroxide shampoo or a very mild bleach.

The Uses of Temporary Haircoloring

First, a reminder: Temporary color should be used with the same respect with which we use other color products. We can get a little too nonchalant with temporary products, and they can stain overporous hair. So choose your color thoughtfully before using it or handing it over to a client.

There are a select few clients who wear nothing but temporary color, most notably, weekly clients who are still hooked on rinses, but most of the time temporary products are used to enhance semi-, demi-, or permanent haircoloring.

When to use temporary haircoloring:

- **Temporary products can be a first-step into color for the uninitiated (young teenagers, or people who are afraid of color). A colored shampoo or conditioner lends just a bit of a new tone, and it's here today, gone tomorrow.**
- **Colored styling and finishing products are the toys of haircoloring, designed more for fun, really, than color change—a streak or a cast that you wash off like makeup.**

- **For a corrective client that you just can't get to until tomorrow, a temporary rinse or pigmented shampoo may save the day, from the client's perspective. Most tonal problems or overlightening can be disguised somewhat with temporary haircoloring.**
- **Highlighted, high-lifted, and bleach-and-tone clients may use temporary products between appointments to keep their hair the tone they prefer, either to eliminate yellow or keep their color sunny.**
- **If a client perpetually fades, no matter what, then a good pigmented shampoo or conditioner can help preserve tint, abating fadage and possibly the need for filling or toning.**
- **The custom mixing of colored shampoos has become an important personal service in salons. Few things make a client feel more special than being handed a shampoo or conditioner that you made just for her!**

Semi-Temporary Haircoloring

To create more durable color deposit, and to create more tonal variety, some manufacturers have made **semi-temporary** products that utilize components of both temporary and semi-permanent haircoloring. These products fall between temporary and semi-permanent color, in terms of their chemistry and wearability. They are more than temporary, but less than semi-permanent. A pigmented shampoo or mousse may utilize semi-permanent dyes, and

Haircoloring Products
continued

ammonia, more-intense color pigment. A lightening and coloring system—with or without heat.

Shampoos

Direct dye pigments added to a shampoo base.

Conditioners

Direct dye pigments added to a conditioner.

Botanical Coloring

A hot water mixed, heat-activated all-natural coloring product. No lift—great deposit. Not recommended for gray coverage, except for blending a very small percentage (colors are brighter on gray hair).

Glazes (Color-and-Shine Products)

A gel-like product to intensify color and add shine—usually heat activated.

Clays

Direct color pigment added to a heat-activated clay pack.

Mousses, Gels, Sprays, and Pomades

Temporary and direct dyes added to styling and finishing products for slight tonal changes or special effects.

last considerably longer in the hair than a true temporary product would.

This brings us to a product form that almost defies classification. In the early 1980s, **color-and-shine** products emerged and enjoyed wide popularity. Most were semi-temporary products. These products declined in popularity toward the end of the '80s (many were discontinued) but are currently enjoying a resurgence. Color-and-shine products are among the most difficult of all haircoloring products to categorize, for the following reasons: first, one brand may be much more penetrating than another; second, any use of heat in processing makes these products much longer lasting; and third, how long the color lasts is much influenced by the quality of the hair to which it is applied. One colored glaze may be accurately categorized as semi-temporary, while another might be more tenacious than permanent color ever dreamed of being. This lack of definition scares off some colorists, but, in truth, this type of direct-dye product is highly useful in the salon.

How do you know if the color deposit will wash out in a single shampoo, in a few weeks, or if it will last longer? Begin by asking the company that makes that particular product. But don't expect these types of products to behave the same way on every head of hair; porosity, especially, and how the client maintains her hair, have a lot to do with how much deposit you get and how long it will last.

SEMI-PERMANENT AND DEMI-PERMANENT HAIRCOLORING

Semi-permanent haircoloring products are designed to last haircut to haircut. Shampooing gradually removes semi-permanent haircoloring (more or less) over a period of about four weeks. The mark of a semi-permanent product is gradual, continuous fadage, and an eventual return to the original, natural color of the hair. Natural pigment is unaltered, no lightening occurs—they are **deposit-only colors.**

The term *semi-permanent* may have always represented something of a misnomer, as it suggests to the client that the artificial coloring will indeed wash out in a limited number of shampoos. Many of these products linger longer than the expected duration, creating an apparently (or truly) permanent deposit of artificial color. So it may be that the name of this category has always been a little misleading. Nonetheless, it is the name we have!

Further complicating matters have been the modern, oxidizing semi-permanents which borrow from the chemistry of permanent haircoloring (we now call these **demi-permanents**), and certain products that are less than semi-permanent, but not really temporary (sometimes called semi-temporary color). But this diversity doesn't have to be confusing. Manufacturers are quite clear about what their products will and will not do. Diversity means versatility! There is a place, a purpose, and a clientele for all of these products.

The Semi-Permanents

True, conventional semi-permanents are simple stains which require no developing agent. The dyes of semi-permanents are called **direct dyes,** or **preformed dyes,** because they color the hair directly, without developer. These direct dye molecules are already fully formed, unlike the dye molecules of permanent haircoloring. Semi-permanent products color the hair without an oxidation process, simply staining the cuticle and, to some degree, the cortex.

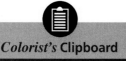

Colorist's Clipboard

Temporary haircoloring:

- *Shampoos out, completely or almost completely, in a single shampoo.*

- *Includes most pigmented shampoos, conditioners, rinses, and styling products.*

- *Some "temporary" products borrow from the chemistry of semi-permanent haircoloring and will last longer in the hair; these are more aptly called semi-temporary products.*

Direct dyes are small enough to penetrate the cuticle, but are much larger than the indirect dyes of permanent haircoloring. Because most clients are multiporous, a combination of **smaller-** and **higher-weight dyes** are used to compensate for the differences in porosity in the average head of hair. This results in more even color than the earliest semi-permanents produced. The labels of semi-permanent products may list disperse dyes, HC dyes, nitro dyes, or acid dyes.

Semi-permanent haircoloring is self-penetrating, relying on natural absorption to enter the hair. Where the hair is more porous, it becomes more stained. These products are usually **alkaline,** which increases absorption by softening and swelling the hair somewhat. Heat processing may be used to increase penetration. Some form of pretreatment or post-treatment may be used to open the cuticle or bind dyes to the hair.

Semi-permanents are completely incapable of lightening and do wash out over time, though perhaps not entirely. Porosity greatly affects both the intensity and duration of color deposit. The degree and duration of deposit depends on the condition of the hair—texture, tenacity, or porosity (more porosity, more deposit)—and on what happens to the hair when the client leaves the salon (mainly what shampoo is used and how often it is used).

The Demi-Permanents

We have continuously demanded more from semi-permanents—more coverage, more durability, more tones, and more evenness of deposit (less porosity-sensitivity)—and manufacturers have responded to these needs by hybridizing the product categories. Demi-permanents are now a category unto themselves: halfway between the semi-permanent and permanent categories, partly belonging to each. These are "semi-permanents" with a developer.

Many modern "semi-permanents" are really oxidation products. **Oxidation haircoloring,** or **oxidative haircoloring** oxidizes, or combines with oxygen, as it processes. When the preparation of haircoloring involves mixing two parts together (this includes crystals, powders, tablets, any packaged liquid or cream additives, and sometimes even water), you are almost certainly creating an oxidation tint. These products contain **indirect dyes** (aniline-derived **intermediates** or **precursors**), once characteristic of only permanent color.

Most demi-permanents may be considered no-lift permanent haircoloring. The advantages of this category over conventional semi-permanents may include greater penetration, more deposit and coverage, natural appearance, longer duration, more intensity, and less porosity-sensitivity. But there may be disadvantages, too: increased porosity, more demarcation and the commitment it poses, and possible lightening of natural pigment.

Oxidation products *do not necessarily lighten natural pigment,* but if that should occur, then that product really has crossed over the line into permanent haircoloring. Obviously, lightening is permanent. No product that lightens hair can be considered anything but permanent haircoloring.

The Semi-Temporaries

Another cousin of the semi-permanents is what might be called semi-temporary color. These products fall between temporary and semi-permanent color, in terms of their chemistry and durability. They use dyes characteristic of both

Semi-permanents are completely incapable of lightening and do wash out over time.

Carole Lyden Smith

owner, Carole Lyden Smith Academy
of Design in Gatlinburg, Tennessee,
on semi-permanent haircoloring:

"Ask your client, 'Would you like

to have shinier, fuller, healthier-

looking hair?'

"What is she going to say?

" 'No, I want my hair to be dry,

dull, damaged and lifeless?!

Mousy / brassy / flat / faded /

and no shine, please!'

"Not likely!"

the temporary and the semi-permanent categories. They may include product forms usually considered temporary (pigmented shampoos or mousses), as well as translucent shine-and-color products.

Remember, the primary defining characteristic of the haircoloring categories is duration—how long the color change lasts. But not all semi-permanent products are created equal. Particularly intense or penetrating direct dyes may stain hair permanently. The processing method makes a difference, too; heat is a catalyst. Heat lifts the cuticle, drives color molecules deeper into the hair, and can fasten dyes more permanently onto the structures of the hair.

Uses of Semi-Temporary, Semi-Permanent, and Demi-Permanent Haircoloring

Semi-permanent haircoloring was first conceived to blend gray, and this continues to be its foremost use. Semi-permanents are ideally suited to this task because they only *deposit* color. A client who just wants to hide a sprinkle of gray does not need lightening and does not necessarily need the penetration of permanent coloring, but she does need more deposit than temporary products offer.

Semi-permanents typically blend low percentages of gray, while demi-permanents blend or cover more gray. Many demi-permanent products are capable of total gray coverage, up to certain percentages. A red or gold semi- or demi-permanent gives the effect of a highlighting on a client whose 20 or 30 percent gray is evenly distributed, brightening the pigmented hair as well. Pale ash colors are often used to whiten gray hair, for clients who like their gray. Light semi-permanent shades can be used on high percentages of gray to tone it blondish.

Semi-permanents are frequently used to introduce clients to color because of the fadage factor (she isn't locked into the service). Semi-permanents tint a little, to ease a client into haircoloring, and demi-permanents tint more, for greater longevity.

These categories lend themselves to numerous corrective uses. Both semi- and demi-permanents may be used to eliminate unwanted casts, deepen lightened ends, tone washed-out highlights, blend excessive highlights, blend uneven color, and refresh faded color. Many make great color fillers. Many demi-permanents produce more even color on multiporous hair than does permanent haircoloring. (Consult manufacturers' literature about the uses of specific brands.)

A client who is allergic to permanent haircoloring can often wear true semi-permanent haircoloring. Proper patch testing is necessary to determine individual sensitivities, of course.

Almost anyone who enters the salon can wear **deposit-only haircoloring.** Most semi- and demi-permanents have a "conditioning" effect, shining and bulking-up the hair. What client would turn down the chance to have shinier, fuller hair? Everybody wants shine! That word—*shine*—is a client hot-button.

Semi-Permanent Haircoloring and Demarcations
No matter what its chemistry, a haircoloring product will create a demarcation if the color change lasts long enough for the hair to grow very much.

Four weeks after her color service, a semi-permanent client will have a **demarcation** to whatever extent the artificial pigment is still in her hair, and to the extent that it is different from her natural pigment. The more the remaining artificial pigment contrasts with the new growth, the more noticeable the demarcation. The higher the percentage of gray, the more noticeable the demarcation.

Darker levels contrast more with a gray new growth. Blond haircoloring on gray hair doesn't appear to "grow out" as soon as brown does because it's not such a stark contrast. The colorist decides whether the client should have more depth and coverage, with its accompanying demarcation, or a lighter blend without the obvious demarcation.

Depending on the client, fadage can either be an advantage or a disadvantage. If a client wants it to gradually fade off, then it's an advantage because there's less commitment. If the client wants a lasting tonal change, lasting depth, or lasting gray coverage, however, then a demi-permanent with real sticking power or permanent haircoloring is more suitable.

PERMANENT HAIRCOLORING

Permanent haircoloring products are designed to permanently alter the natural pigmentation of hair.

The permanence of these products has two facets. The primary defining characteristic of permanent haircoloring is that it is capable of lightening natural pigment. Ammonia, or another catalyst in the dye-bearing liquid, gel, or cream, combines with hydrogen peroxide in the developer to lighten natural pigment. Hence, the change is permanent.

The secondary facet of permanence is penetration. Permanent haircoloring is designed for penetration—ammonia to soften and swell the cuticle, promoting penetration, and tiny dye molecules, sized to penetrate. This ability to fully penetrate and color the cuticle and cortex is so important that perma-

nent haircoloring products were originally also called **penetrating tints.**

Though very unlike other permanent haircoloring, vegetable dyes (including **henna**) and **metallic dyes** were originally grouped in this category. The action of henna and metallics is coating as well as penetrating, since neither is capable of lightening, and it was due to their wearability alone that they were considered permanent products. Their chemistry is completely different from **aniline-derivative tints.** If henna had been discovered by a company in the 1990s instead of by the ancients, it would be sold as the latest, greatest, long-wearing semi-permanent. Its categorization as a permanent haircoloring is an anomaly by today's standards. A pure henna product has a place in the professional dispensary (it is generally nonallergenic and has a certain "natural" appeal), but metallics, of course, do not (metallic salts are incompatible with oxidative chemicals).

Today, the term *permanent haircoloring* really refers exclusively to oxidation tints capable of lift.

How Permanent Haircoloring Works

Permanent haircoloring has two aspects: lightening, and penetrating, permanent deposit. All permanent haircoloring products work about the same. To date, there are few significant variations.

The ability of permanent haircoloring to lighten natural pigment comes from two key ingredients: the **ammonia,** or other **catalyst,** in the dye-containing liquid, gel, or cream, and the hydrogen peroxide in the developer. It is the combination of the two that creates lift.

Ammonia is a critical ingredient in permanent haircoloring. A permanent haircoloring

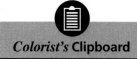

Colorist's Clipboard

- *The preparation of semi-permanent haircoloring does not involve mixing. True semi-permanents contain only direct dyes which do not require a developer.*

- *Demi-permanents are mixed with a developing agent because they contain oxidation dyes.*

- *Some products borrow from the chemistry of both temporary and semi-permanent haircoloring and are more aptly called semi-temporary.*

Hydrogen Peroxide Percent and Volume Equivalencies

Developer strength is sometimes expressed in percent rather than volume.

- 3% hydrogen peroxide is the same as 10 volume;
- 6% is the same as 20 volume;
- 9% is the same as 30 volume, and
- 12% is the same as 40 volume.

product always contains ammonia, or another base that does what ammonia does. Too much ammonia is unnecessarily damaging but, without ammonia, penetration, lightening, and dye development would not occur. It, or something like it, is essential.[1] Manufacturers of professional products strive to put just enough—and not too much—ammonia in their permanent haircoloring.

Ammonia is an **alkali;** it swells the hair shaft, promoting penetration. It is also a catalyst, and this is its primary purpose: to facilitate lightening by releasing oxygen, supplied by the developer, to oxidize natural pigment. Ammonia, lastly, creates the necessary alkalinity for the development of permanent dyes; permanent haircoloring is always alkaline in **pH.**

The ammonia of a haircoloring product is not in the developer; it is in the bottle or tube

with the dyes. Higher (lighter) levels contain more ammonia than lower (darker) levels, in order to provide more lightening capability. When you mix the lightest levels in your system, you smell much more ammonia than when you mix the darkest levels.

The higher the level, the more ammonia (lift) and the less pigment (deposit). The lower the level, the less lift and the greater the deposit. That's why a medium blond will cover gray better than a very light blond. It is also why a medium brown will not lift as many levels as high-lift tint.

High-lift colors contain the most ammonia, to have the most aggressive and extended lift cycles. That much ammonia in darker levels, however, would be overkill. Ammonia is calibrated (graduated) by level in all professional products.

Another critical component of permanent haircoloring is hydrogen peroxide.[2] The devel-

---

1 *A common ammonia substitute is monoethanolamine, also called MEA. It, like ammonia, is an alkali. It and other ethanolamines are used to elevate the pH of haircoloring in the same way and for the same purpose as ammonia.*

Permanent dyes have been demonstrated to work satisfactorily using certain enzymes (e.g., uricase and glucose oxidase) which activate oxygen in the air to accomplish oxidation with lower volumes of hydrogen peroxide.

---

2 *A few oxidizing products use crystals or powders as oxidizers rather than liquid or cream hydrogen peroxide. These all consist of peroxides or superoxides in powder form.*

One form of oxidizing tint, novel in the USA but more common in other countries, consists of dry dyes and oxidizer in one blended powder, which is shaken with water.

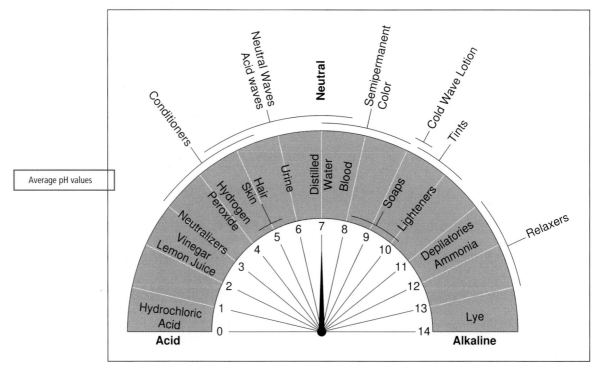

Average pH values

opers for permanent haircoloring products, whether clear or cream, are hydrogen peroxide. **Hydrogen peroxide** is the oxidizer of permanent haircoloring, providing the oxygen for lightening of natural pigment, and for the development of artificial pigment. Permanent haircoloring is sometimes also called oxidation or oxidative haircoloring. It is the hydrogen peroxide in permanent haircoloring—not the ammonia—that causes oxidative hair damage. Good colorists are aware of the damage created by excessively high developer volumes and utilize only that which is necessary.

The chemical "shorthand" for hydrogen peroxide, H_2O_2, means "Two hydrogen atoms and two oxygen atoms." Higher volumes of hydrogen peroxide provide more oxygen for more extended lightening. *Higher volumes create more lift and less deposit; lower volumes create less lift and greater deposit.* This is why better gray coverage is achieved with 20 volume rather than 40 volume (with some products, 10 or 15 volume may be even better), and it is why the same level red tint on the same natural base will be brighter and clearer with a higher volume, and deeper and richer with a lower volume.

Some strength of hydrogen peroxide has to be used in order to develop the dyes of permanent haircoloring. Just to get the dyes to color the hair, an oxidizer has to be present. (And peroxide all by itself won't lighten the hair, either. It needs to react with ammonia in order for efficient oxidation to occur.) Peroxide, ammonia, and the dyes all need each other to get the haircoloring to work.

The dyes in permanent haircoloring, all aniline derivatives or aniline relatives (aromatic amines) of various types, are mainly indirect dyes, which must undergo oxidation in order to color the hair. These are also called **dye precursors,** or intermediates. The **dye intermediates** are tiny, colorless dye molecules that develop into large, colored molecules when oxidized. Hydrogen peroxide is required as an oxidizer, or developer.

Shortly after the dye-bearing liquid, gel, or cream is combined with the hydrogen peroxide developer, dye molecules begin developing, rearranging into bigger, complex, colored molecules. That's the reason haircoloring should not be mixed until just before application—that, and the fact that the lift cycle is underway soon after mixing. Color deposit and lifting capability begin ticking away about ten minutes after the colorant is mixed with the developer, giving the stylist 10 or 15 minutes of application time.

The tiny size of the dye precursors before oxidation enables them to pass easily into the cortex of the hair, penetrating it fully. As the color processes, the tiny dye molecules change structure, coupling up to form big, colored molecules. These newly created dye molecules, now too big to leave the hair the way they came in, affix themselves to the keratin chains in the hair.

Permanent haircoloring always uses oxidation dyes; these include **paraphenylenediamine, paratoulenediamine, metaphenylenediamine, paraaminophenol,** and numerous others. Permanent haircoloring may also contain direct, preformed dyes, which is why it may be yellow, red, or violet straight from the tube or bottle (before oxidation).

The use of permanent haircoloring always results in a line of demarcation. How greatly the natural color was altered (how different the formula was from her natural color) determines how distinct the demarcation is.

Uses of Permanent Haircoloring

If you or I could have only one haircoloring product to work with, it would have to be permanent haircoloring: A good colorist can make permanent haircoloring do almost any-

Dr. Leszek J. Wolfram

cosmetic chemist, on the effect of hydrogen peroxide on hair structure:

"H_2O_2, particularly in aggressive formulations used in bleaching, breaks considerable numbers of disulfide cross-links causing so-called oxidative hair damage. When permanent dyes are used, the frequency of the process leads to cumulative hair damage, as the latter cannot be repaired. Thus, although care is taken to limit and mask the damage [I must] stress its existence . . .

"Often, because of its odor, ammonia is picked on as the culprit in hair damage. Nonsense!"

thing necessary. Some colorists even prefer this. Most would agree, though, that specialized products do specialized jobs best—that is, the best temporary or semi-permanent services are done with temporary or semi-permanent dye products.

Permanent haircoloring is the only category capable of lightening natural pigment. How many of your color clients want to be lighter than their natural base? That's how important this category is.

The brightest reds and golds are achieved with permanent haircoloring, as is the most perfect gray coverage. By far, the great majority of corrective and creative coloring is done with permanent products. This is the category that best meets the needs of the majority of clients.

Colorist's Clipboard

Temporary haircoloring:
- *Lasts shampoo to shampoo.*
- *Includes most colored shampoos, conditioners, styling products, etc.*
- *Color deposit is superficial (lays on the cuticle).*
- *Is deposit only.*

Semi-temporary haircoloring:
- *Lasts longer than conventional temporary color (contains some semi-permanent dyes).*
- *Includes some colored shampoos, mousses and some color-and-shine products.*
- *Is deposit only.*

Semi-permanent haircoloring:
- *Lasts haircut to haircut.*
- *Direct dyes, no developer required, no mixing.*
- *Incapable of lightening; deposit only.*

Demi-permanent haircoloring:
- *Uses oxidation dyes, requires a developer.*
- *Usually deposit only, but some can lighten natural pigment.*

- *More penetrating and longer-lasting than semi-permanent color.*

Permanent haircoloring:
- *Uses oxidation dyes; requires a developer.*
- *Capable of lightening natural pigment.*
- *Developer volume is varied to increase or decrease lightening.*

Vegetable (botanical or plant) dyes:
- *Henna and hennalike products.*
- *Incapable of lightening.*
- *Most fade minimally and are therefore classified as "permanent."*

Color-and-Shine Glazes:
- *Deposit only.*
- *Fadage varies; it may be rapid and almost complete (semi-temporary), or it may be minimal (stong colors, especially when heat-processed, may stain the hair permanently).*

part two

2

the universal method of formulation

The chief concern stylists have about haircoloring is knowing how to formulate: What do I use to get the color I want? Without a method, you are reduced to guessing—trial and error—which is a pretty lost feeling. If you formulate methodically, though, you are insulated from most errors as you develop your coloring skills, like how partings made before the cut help keep the cutter out of trouble. Advance planning is what good formulation is all about: Plan your work, Work your plan; Work Smart.

Eventually, the method you practice becomes second nature, like breathing.

Knowledge of basic theory provides the groundwork for formulation skills. Proper formulation is based entirely on universal haircoloring principles, specific product knowledge, and good client communication.

A good formula, using any product, and for any client, always considers the same set of variables: This set consists of natural base level, percentage of gray, texture, porosity, existing tint, the client's desires, what looks best on her, and what she can maintain. These are the variables that determine every successful formula, no matter who is formulating or what product is being formulated.

The only sure way to get perfect results is to consider all the relevant variables beforehand, communicate carefully with the client, and target the end result precisely. And that is, in fact, the **Universal Method of Formulation.**

The Universal Method enables colorists to rapidly master different haircoloring products. This does *not* mean that we do not have to read manufacturer's directions. On the contrary, there is no substitute for a careful reading of all directions! No amount of general knowledge can replace the specific information companies provide about their products.

The Universal Method applies equally to new and returning color clients. Although the consultation for a returning client is more brief—usually much more brief—than for a new color client, it should not be entirely skipped, because the client's needs may change and her hair may change, as well.

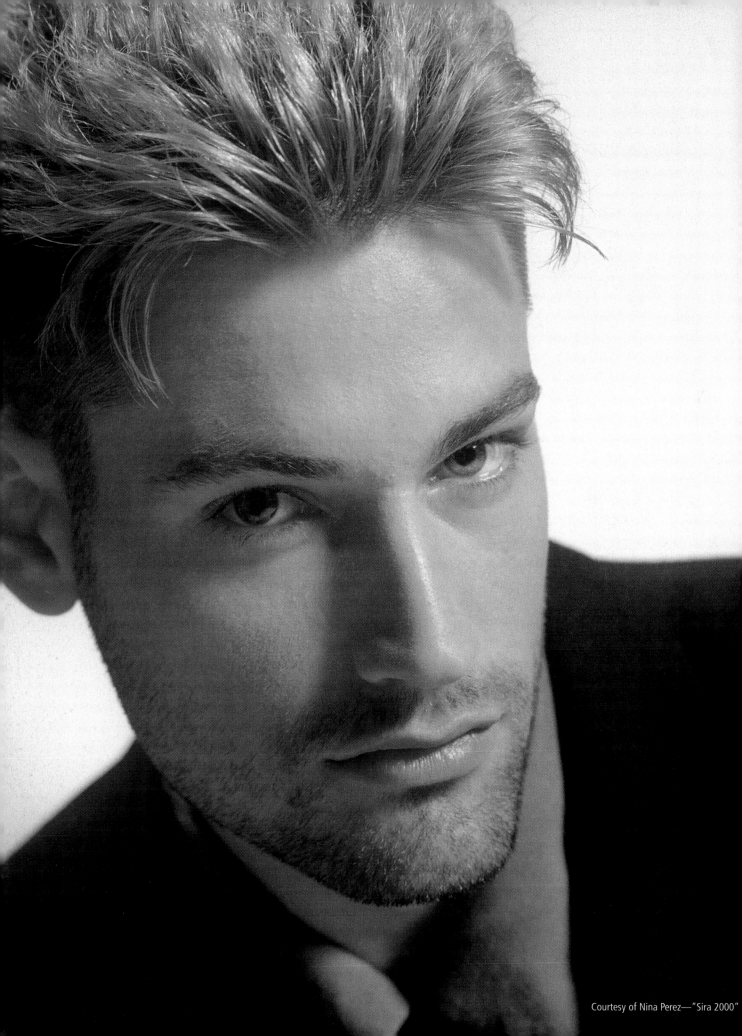

chapter four

analyzing the hair

When you formulate, you first analyze the factors that are going to affect the final color result. This is crucial. To skip this is to mix color blindfolded. The key factors that affect a haircoloring result are: natural base level, percentage of gray, texture, porosity, and existing tint.

This text is more oriented toward permanent haircoloring as, industry-wide, more permanent haircoloring is used than any other type, but the principles of formulation apply to all categories of color. Omit any talk of lightening or developer selection, and the guidelines are essentially the same for nonlift products.

The Key Factors and Ethnic Background

Although wide variation exists within groups, ethnic background does lend certain characteristics to hair. African-American hair tends to be very curly, and darker and coarser, on average, than Caucasian hair. Caucasian hair tends to be lighter in color and finer in texture than that of other ethnic groups. Asian hair tends to be coarse, resistant, very dark, and very straight.

But the basic structure of hair does not vary group to group—it is the same for all of humanity. Whether it is curly or straight, the same rules apply when it comes to haircoloring. All hair is analyzed in the same way, because the same variables always affect the color result.

1. **NATURAL BASE LEVEL.** *How dark the hair is to start with essentially determines how light it can be made in a single process.* Knowing the natural base level also enables you to select the proper developer strength. And natural level tells you what kind of underlying color tone you are dealing with: Will it enhance the final result, or must you formulate to contrast it out? (Dominant underlying color, also known as **contributing pigment, natural underlying pigment, undertones,** and so forth, is automatically considered when natural base level is identified, but it is sometimes emphasized as a separate factor.)

2. **PERCENTAGE OF GRAY.** Gray hair is basically unpigmented. Artificial pigment looks different on gray or white hair because of its lack of depth and lack of underlying warmth. An ash formula on gray hair will not cover the gray, a brilliant red will appear garish, and so on. All manufacturers recommend specific adjustments for high percentages of gray. Some products are designed to fully cover gray, while others only blend it.

3. **TEXTURE.** Fine hair processes faster, lightens more, and tends to show more of the tone and depth of the formula. Coarse hair takes longer to penetrate and lighten and may require a stronger developer. Coarse hair has more underlying pigment, which is more difficult to contrast-out.

4. **POROSITY.** Tenacious (resistant) hair is slower to accept haircoloring and may require a stronger developer and longer processing (and possibly presoftening). Overporous hair processes quickly, and may require more warmth in the formula and a weaker developer (and possibly prepigmenting).

5. **EXISTING TINT.** As a rule, going lighter than existing tint requires **decolorizing** (color removal).

HOW TO ASSESS THE KEY FACTORS

It takes about one minute to evaluate the key factors that will affect the color result. Of the time that goes into a haircoloring service, this one minute may be the most vital. Your formula will be only as good as your analysis. Factor in the wrong information, and you will get the wrong result. (In computerese, GIGO— **G**arbage **I**n, **G**arbage **O**ut!) It is not difficult to do a good analysis; you just have to know what to look for.

You have greeted your client and let her talk a little about her hair; now you tell her you need a moment to look at her hair. Make notes as you do so. When it comes time to actually formulate, it is helpful to have this information on paper, in front of you.

1. IDENTIFYING THE CLIENT'S NATURAL BASE LEVEL (HOW LIGHT OR HOW DARK THE CLIENT IS TO START WITH). Natural level is always "read" at the scalp area, because hair is always lighter on the length and ends, even on a virgin head. Part the hair down to the scalp. Don't press her hair flat to her head; hair appears darker without light filtering through. Gently push her hair up alongside the part line, lifting it just slightly. Check in front, in back, at the crown, at the nape, around the ears. Occasionally a client's level is considerably different in different areas of her head. (This is why you really can't check your own natural level.)

The most foolproof way to identify natural base level is to directly compare the client's hair to **synthetic swatches.** Most manufacturers provide removable swatches or a swatch ring for this purpose. If you do have loose or detachable swatches, by all means use them.

Loose swatches are not available in all systems, however, in which case natural level is identified by indirect comparison. This takes a trained eye. Your eye is trained by studying the manufacturer's swatchbook. Thoroughly familiarize yourself with the neutral (natural) series swatches, committing to memory the lightness or depth of each level. Do not study a **paper chart;** they are not accurate. Refer to the synthetic swatches as you examine your client's hair. You may be able to lay her hair on the swatchbook, but remember that *base level is read at the scalp area,* not on the midshaft or ends.

Ask yourself: Is the client light, medium, or dark? Select a swatch in the appropriate range. Fan the swatch slightly, to resemble the natural density of your client's hair, but don't splay it out so much that you are comparing two synthetic fibers to 20 natural hairs. The purpose of fanning the swatch is to duplicate natural density—natural hair is not as dense as a swatch; our follicles just aren't that close together.

Part the client's hair down to the scalp. Gently push the hair up to allow light to diffuse through it. Lay the slightly fanned swatch against her new growth, so that light strikes the swatch and her hair at the same angle.

If the swatch almost seems to disappear into her hair, that's her natural base level. You have a match when you can hardly tell where the hair leaves off and the swatch begins. If the swatch stands out against the background of her natural hair, then it doesn't match; try another.

Sometimes a client's natural level will fall between levels, between a 5 level and a 6 level, for instance. If you are lightening (and most clients go lighter), then designate her the darker of the two: a 5 level. In this way, you avoid underlightening her and getting a too-warm, too-deep result. (Note: If you have just changed product lines, remember that the level systems of different manufacturers differ somewhat—a light brown may be a 6 in one system and a 5 in another—double check your work until the system is second nature to you.)

Identification of natural level is usually done by comparison to neutral series swatches because most people are naturally neutral in tone. This is not always the case, however. Hair that is naturally red is compared to the manufacturer's red-brown or red-blond swatches, or sometimes the golden series swatches. Some people are naturally very ash, in which case you refer to the manufacturer's ash series. Here is a hint to help you recognize ash hair: ashy hair reflects less light and therefore appears less shiny; it may appear dull or flat, or lack sparkle.

Natural level is always read on dry hair. (Damp hair looks darker. Soiled or oily hair looks darker, too.)

Be extra-vigilant when lighting is different or imperfect—at night or in a different area of the salon. Use the best available lighting to do color consultations. Indirect natural light, or its artificial equivalent, is the ideal.

Colorist's **Clipboard**

The five key factors that affect the color result:

- Natural base level
- Percentage of gray
- Texture
- Porosity (condition)
- Existing tint

A misreading of natural base level will throw the formula off, yielding an unanticipated result. The same formula on different base levels yields different results. You can put the same formula on six different bases and get six different results! Take care to do a good reading.

2. IDENTIFYING PERCENTAGE OF GRAY. As you are checking natural base level, also look for gray. If she has gray, estimate the percentage.

Remember this rule of thumb: if your first impression is gray, she is over 50 percent; if your first impression is her natural level, she is under 50 percent. Decide if she is over, under, or right at 50 percent gray.

"10 percent gray" means that one out of ten hairs is gray—not a lot, but enough to really affect how she looks and feels—and "25 percent" means that one out of four hairs is gray. Now don't go counting hairs! You are *estimating,* not *computing.* Just form an impression of whether the gray is a small minority (5 to 15 percent), a large minority (25 or 30 percent), salt and pepper (40 to 60 percent), or an overwhelming majority (75 to 80 percent); 90 percent looks practically solid white.

Percentage of gray is not normally uniform all over the head. Clients are usually grayer in front and darker in back. This may present an opportunity to achieve a bit of a dimensional result. With many products, if you use the same formula all over, she will be slightly lighter in front—a natural and desirable variance. A single formula on uneven gray usually creates minor, natural variations in level or tone. With high-coverage, opaque-finish products, however, there is rarely a detectable variation at all.

Every so often a client's pattern of gray makes it necessary to use two formulas—one for where the percentage is high (the facial hairline, usually), one for darker areas (in the crown, for instance). Spot pretreatment may be necessary if gray is very spotty. These are atypical cases, but they do occur.

3. IS THERE ANYTHING UNUSUAL ABOUT THE TEXTURE OF THE HAIR? Is the hair unusually coarse? Unusually fine? Most people have average (medium) texture, which demands no special consideration.

For extremely fine or extremely coarse hair, you may have to alter the formula, processing time, and/or application. The developer chosen, the amount of ash in the formula, timing, and application all may be influenced by texture, so anything out of the ordinary should be noted. Nine times out of ten, texture is average and normal and does not affect the formula.

There are two common textural aberrations: an ultrafine hairline which will accept color very quickly (decrease timing by applying color to the hairline last), and ultracoarse hair which is harder to penetrate and lift (increase timing and anticipate greater natural warmth).

4. IS THERE ANYTHING UNUSUAL ABOUT THE POROSITY OF THE HAIR? Normal porosity means a slightly raised cuticle—just barely lifted. For normal hair, you formulate normally; no adjustments. The majority of clients have normal porosity.

Second-most-common is multiporosity: overporous ends, with a normal scalp area and midshaft. The more overporous the ends are, the more the formula, application, and timing must be adjusted, the more quickly the

Use the best available lighting to do color consultations.

hair will process, and the more it will tend to pick up drab tones. Strand-testing is the best way to determine exactly what adjustments are necessary.

Overporous hair is damaged. It *looks* rough, dull, perhaps lightened or faded. It *feels* rough: the cuticle scales are lifted, ruffled, open.

On the other end of the spectrum is tenacious, or resistant, hair. Tenacious hair is glassy and smooth. It looks and feels slick, because it is slick—the cuticle is very compact. Gray hair is often resistant, as is coarse hair; it takes longer to penetrate and may require a somewhat stronger developer.

5. IS THERE ANY ARTIFICIAL PIGMENT ALREADY IN THE HAIR? The presence of artificial haircoloring is detected by observation and questioning. Take care in your inquiry, however. If you ask, "Do you have any artificial color on your hair?" she may not tell you about the semi-permanent color she used a few months ago because she thinks it's gone.

Instead, ask: "Have you had your hair colored, or put any color on your hair, within the last year or so? I need to know all about your hair, and about your experiences with color."

Observation reveals a lot as well. Look for unevenness of level, bands, or demarcations. Hold up thin sections of hair and view them from scalp to ends. Virgin hair will appear either even or naturally graduated. If there are any signs of haircoloring, let her know that any previous chemical will affect today's service. If her length appears sunlightened, tell her it is important that you know about the presence of any foreign substance: Did she put something on her hair to promote lightening?

If the client does have artificial color on her hair, the next step is to *identify the level of the existing tint.* Use the manufacturer's swatches to do this.

a. If the existing tint is significantly lighter than the desired end result, you may need to prepigment (fill) where the hair is too light.

b. If the existing tint is the same level as what she wants (or not much more than a level lighter) and similar in tone, then no extra steps are necessary. Your formula will simply blend and cover it.

c. If the existing tint is darker than what she wants, you will first have to lighten it (color removal or decolorizing). And if the existing tint is much redder or browner than what she wants, even though it isn't darker, it also requires some removal. As a general rule, *artificial tint does not lift artificial tint;* it is designed to lighten only natural pigment.

The method of removal depends on the haircoloring product to be removed, so *find out what was used.* Find out the brand name if at all possible, especially if it was a semi-permanent. Permanent haircoloring products are all removed in much the same way, but the semi-permanents are another story, and some "semi-permanent" stains are very difficult to lift.

Neither prepigmenting nor decolorizing is as difficult as you may think. If you are afraid of either, after you have done it a few times you will wonder why you were ever afraid!

CONCLUSION

Greet and seat your client. After relaxing her with your ice-breaking conversation and listening ear, tell her you are now going to analyze her hair. Do so, quickly and accurately. Take notes. Explain your analysis only as necessary and in general terms.

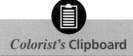

Colorist's **Clipboard**

Analyzing the hair before color

• Write down the answers to these questions:

1. What is her natural base level?

2. Percentage of gray?

3. Is she unusually fine or coarse?

4. Is her hair resistant? Overporous (damaged)?

5. Is there any artificial coloring already on her hair? What is it, and what level is it?

A good analysis should be brief and methodical. The client doesn't have to know specifically what you are doing; she only knows you are assessing her hair. Remember, the key factors that affect the haircoloring result are the same regardless of product or ethnicity. First, identify her natural base level. Next, does she have gray, and if so, how much? Then, is there anything unusual about the texture or condition (porosity) of her hair?

Finally, find out about any artificial coloring already present.

That's it.

The most important of these key factors is often natural level, but don't take the others for granted. All of the key factors affect the final result and will shape how you proceed: how you formulate, how you apply, and the processing time you allow.

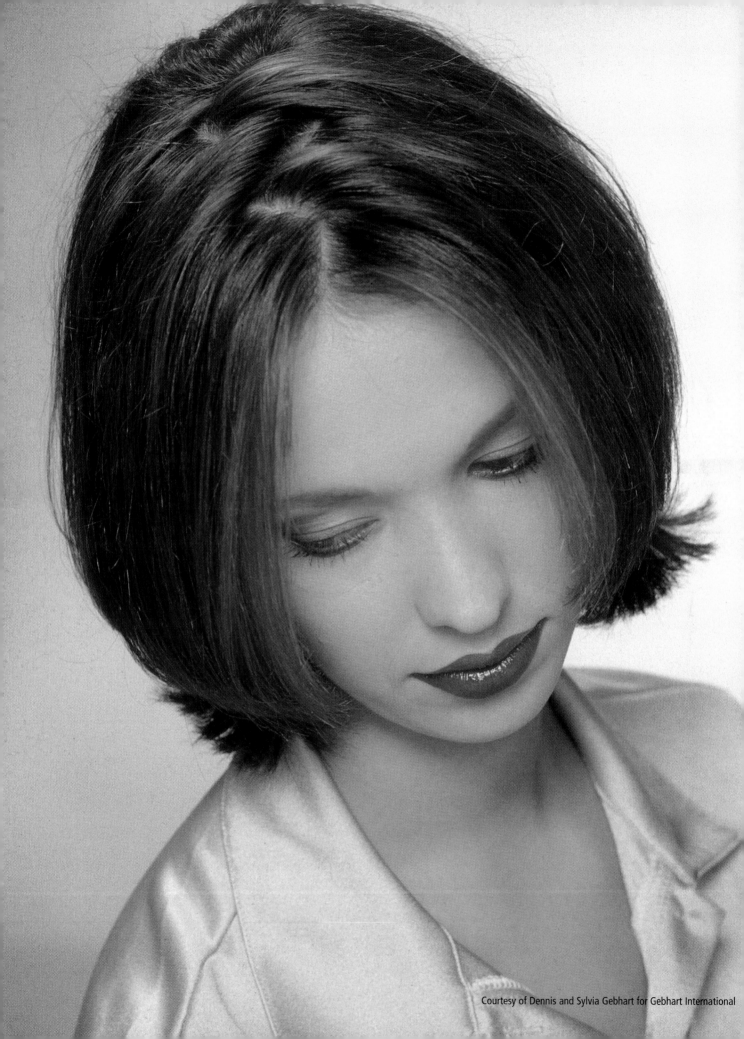

chapter five

communicating with the client

Communication begins, of course, the moment the client walks into the salon (or before, on the phone). The seconds spent greeting a client often reveal what you will be doing today. Clients very often echo your "good morning" and then launch right into what they want.

Once the hair has been analyzed, you can then repeat back to the client her initial remarks, and advise her.

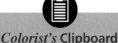

Colorist's Clipboard

What does the client want? What is she thinking about her color?

- Listen for clues.

- Look for clues.

- Ask for clues.

Have her show you what she wants.

CHANGING THE NATURAL COLOR

Natural base level is the jumping-off point for all haircoloring consultations. How can you discuss change, after all, if you don't know what you are changing?

Permanent haircoloring can only lighten so much. Unless bleach is used, a client is limited to a certain range of lightness by her natural level, usually four levels lighter. By identifying natural level, you determine the limits of lightness for that client, so if the client wants to be much lighter than she is naturally, you can tell her exactly what is possible without bleach.

If the client says she wants to be her natural color, you can show her exactly what her natural color is. It may surprise her! Most clients think they are lighter than they actually are, because hair is always a little lighter on the ends (and tends to be lighter in front).

The more gray a client has, the lighter she perceives herself. It is almost never appropriate to return a client with a high percentage of gray to her original depth. Be careful in your selection of desired level for a gray or graying client!

Natural base level also tells you what is likely to appear most natural to a client. Going more than two levels lighter than natural level, or going at all darker, is a dramatic change. Of course, drama may be just what she's after! Men rarely want dramatic changes. Natural-looking options are **highlighting** or **multi-shading,** or matching or going a little lighter than the natural base.

There are only three possible variations on natural color (or existing tint):

- *Lighter*
- *Darker*
- *A different tone*

Find out what level the client is naturally; ask her what she has been thinking about her color. Listen and advise.

THE CLIENT'S PREFERENCES

Whatever the client wants, of course, really *is* the desired end result!

Most clients don't have too much trouble telling you what they want. All visual aids should be welcomed—magazines, style books, photos, wigs, friends, swatches, whatever. Visuals are invaluable when it comes to client communication. Something you can both look at helps to ensure that you and your client understand one another. Another good tool is a **color album** (an assortment of good colors and special effects from magazines, or your own photography).

Visuals give the client a way to clearly express what she has in mind, and also give you a way to show the client what objectively suits her. You can use a thousand words to describe a color and still not be sure your client is thinking what you are thinking! Words like *wheat, champagne, platinum,* and even *light brown* may paint totally different pictures in your mind and in your client's mind. Color just has to be *seen!*

Most clients desire subtlety—neutral tones or a little gold or auburn. Some people are attracted to warm tones, some to cool tones. Same with depth; some people are most at home in light colors, some in medium colors, some in deep colors. Many people are very definite about their preferences, and are quite correct about what looks best on them. Others are confused by the whole business and rely more heavily on their colorist's advice.

Observe your client's makeup, nail color, and clothing. This will give you an idea of what she likes. Most of the time you won't have to ask her about her preferences; she will begin telling you before she even sits down! The first thing she says will usually be what is most important to her: "Don't make me orange!" / "I'm tired of always seeing roots." / "My hair is so dull!" / "I hate my gray!" / "This color makes me feel all washed out!" / "Don't you think I'm too light (dark)?" / "I want it to look natural."

Some clients are more reserved with their opinions. Open-ended questions—questions you can't answer with just "yes" or "no"—help get the consultation up and running. Kay Nielsen, owner of Scruples Hair Design in Roswell, Georgia, used to ask clients: "If you could be any color in the world, any color at all, what color would you chose?" Other openers are:

- "Show me what you like."
- "Show me what you don't like."
- "How are you feeling about your color?"
- "What have you been thinking about your hair?"

Leading questions are helpful with the most reticent clients:

- "Were you thinking of going lighter?"
- "How do you like this red?"

Don't ever let a client "leave it up to you." Everyone has an opinion; insist she share hers. If you don't find out what she wants before you color her hair, you can bet you will find out afterwards! Even when clients say, "I don't care," they care! Be sure you are clear about your client's preferences, and be sure she is clear about the level and tone that you settle on together.

Remember that clients don't always ask for appropriate colors; don't agree to give a client the color she requests without first considering if it is really suitable for her. That's where your professional judgment comes in.

If you get a client in your chair who can't make up her mind, allow her a few minutes alone to think it over; otherwise she may tie you up in an endless debate. If she remains undecided, you may have to tell her you feel she is not ready for a change. Coloring a client who can't tell you what she wants is asking for trouble.

PROFESSIONAL OPINION: THE COLORIST'S OBJECTIVE ADVICE

What haircoloring will really be most complimentary? These are the elements that define her options:

a. **Her skin tone and eye color.**
b. **Her personality and lifestyle.**
c. **Her haircut and how she styles it.**

Skin Tone and Eye Color

Good haircoloring enhances skin texture and tone as well as eye color. The right haircoloring makes a person look less plain and more radiant—skin smoother, more even; complexion creamier or more glowing and rosy; eyes brighter and more outstanding. The right haircoloring makes people look healthy, alive, youthful.

Color analysis is based on color wheel theory. Some salons use a sophisticated system of color analysis, but it is not necessary. Almost all stylists were born with an excellent eye for color and are able to recognize whether a client is prettier in warm tones or in cool tones. Do read a book or attend a class on color analysis, but don't make it more time-consuming than it has to be, unless the client is paying you for a color analysis service.

Lee Hoffman

owner of Salon Hudson, Hudson and Cleveland, Ohio:

"Truly listening to what your clients say involves more than hearing the words coming from their mouths. Actively work at listening, so that your mind doesn't wander . . .

"Listen for ideas and clues to each client's likes and dislikes as well as for important details. Write these ideas down as soon as possible so you don't forget them. . .

"Give your clients feedback. Confirm that you hear what your clients are saying by just repeating it back to them in their own words. That way, if there is miscommunication, it can be straightened out before making any mistakes."

—*from* Keep 'Em Coming Back: SalonOvations Guide to Salon Promotion and Client Retention *(Albany, NY: Milady Publishing, 1994), p. 55.*

Lili Jakel

on understanding hair color suitability:

To make a client look good and therefore feel better is the ultimate challenge and responsibility. Knowing this, we must not only learn and educate ourselves, but we must experience, feel, and care for her and her needs.

This can be achieved when we help her make the right choices. Suitability is everything. We must think in terms of working with her skin color (this should be at least 80 percent of the decision making). Eye color makes up the last 20 percent in deciding on the final choice. Natural hair color should be taken into consideration when it is a question of maintenance and budget.

Ultimately it is the individual person who often has an image in mind. This is where our expertise as far as suitability and maintenance makes us the professional hair color expert. The clients of the '90s seek and deserve a professional hair color expert.

Skin tone is usually the most important consideration in selecting the tone of the haircoloring. Look at the client's facial skin (especially the skin of her jawline or her forehead, away from the flush of her cheeks), her neck, and the inside of her forearm, where she is unlikely to be tanned.

A client with a golden or peachy complexion (yellow-orange undertones) looks best in golden blonds, golden browns, or golden reds. Someone whose skin has cool undertones (blue-red or blue-pink) looks best in cool hair, ashes to neutrals to cool reds. This applies to all ethnic groups. For dark skin with red undertones, reddish browns work well; for dark skin with gold undertones, golden browns and dark blonds are good choices.

Skin tone usually determines whether you color the client cool or warm, but **eye color** also plays a role. In fact, for some colorists, eye color is the determining factor. Blue and gray eyes are cool, and usually look most outstanding with cool hair. Warm brown eyes are prettiest with warm hair. Green eyes are neutral, the hair can be either ash or warm. Eyes that are so dark they are almost black are also neutral. When you look at your client's eyes, notice more than just the overall color. Look closely for variations of colors within the eye, warm or cool flecks, and the rim of the iris. For eyes that are green with yellow flecks, for instance, golden highlights are prettier than cool ones.

The easiest way to tell which levels and tones are most complimentary to a client is to hold swatches to her face. (This is also the most effective way to convince her!) Place swatches of different tones and levels near the outer corner of her eye, at her temple. Some colors will flatter her, lighting up her skin and eyes. Others will make her look florid, sallow, "hard," or "washed out." Some will exaggerate flaws in her complexion (blemishes, lines, dark circles); others will seem to erase the imperfections. (Note: If your manufacturer doesn't provide removable swatches, make some of your own. Use hair you've cut, sections about four inches long and pencil-thick. Secure the hairs together at the root end with tape, clear nail polish, glue, or a crimper.[1] Then color the strands and use them to demonstrate different tones. Swatches for coloring can also be purchased.)

The ideal color for a client will make her look better even when she isn't wearing makeup; the wrong color will send her running for her makeup bag. When a client wakes up in the morning and looks in the mirror barefaced, her haircoloring should please her, not startle her.

Some people wear lighter colors best; some, darker colors. Haircoloring should not look harsh—dramatic, perhaps, but not harsh. Youth can generally wear extremes better than age. Too bright and, especially, too light or too dark, is aging; skin that is lined should be softly surrounded.

Hair is a frame for the face. To define the face, haircolor has to contrast with skin color, it has to be either lighter or darker than the skin. If hair and skin are the same level, everything runs together. A color that provides the contrast needed to make her face stand out is usually best, but remember that extreme contrast makes flaws in the skin more pronounced.

1 For detailed instruction on how to make your own swatches, read "Making Swatches for Experiments" in Andre Nizetich's Teaching Hair Coloring: A Step-by-Step Guide to Building Props (Albany, NY: Milady Publishing, 1993), pp. 106–109.

Both extremely light colors and very dark colors exaggerate the sparseness of a fine, thin head of hair. The colors of the medium range (medium brown to medium blond) make fine hair look more substantial.

It is best to establish exactly what the client wants and should have, of course, but if you aren't 100 percent sure, go a little lighter rather than darker. People can usually live with a color that is a tad too light, but if it is too dark, she will hate it! (And better you should have to deepen a little, rather than have to decolorize.)

The Same Art Principles Apply to Everyone

The **principles of color harmony** are the same for light skin, dark skin, and every skin in-between, just as the laws of line, design, balance, and proportion apply universally. Ruth Sinclair of Khamit Kinks, in Atlanta, Georgia, and New York City, learned color harmony from her training in portrait painting:

The skin tone picks up around the upper part of the cheeks, around the eyes, and in the middle of the forehead, the chin . . . In painting, that's where you put the highlight . . . A client with jet black skin may have a reddish tone in those areas and I might color her burgundy, with brown in it—the haircoloring reflects the color of her face.

A lot of black women like light hair but they don't want to be blond. If their skin has yellow undertones, I will use a yellow-brown color—I will look for a yellow base, and then select a brown in that base color. If there is red-yellow in their skin, I use a red with gold in it.

Exceptions to the Rules

Let's review: Clients with warm natural coloring look best in warm hair and clients with cool coloring look best in cool hair; the tone of the hair should agree with the client's skin tone; the level of the hair should contrast with the level of the skin, within a reasonable range.

Those are the rules, and most color services conform to the rules. But be prepared for exceptions.

- **A client may objectively look best in golden colors but strongly prefer cool ones. She won't feel right in what is objectively best for her.**
- **Remember, too, that "cool" and "warm" are relative terms. For a client with naturally ash hair, a neutral tone is relatively warm.**
- **You will have clients who can wear either cool or warm tones, as long as they adjust their makeup and clothing accordingly.**
- **And you may run across a client with cool skin and a bold personality that likes the jarring contrast of orange. Sometimes people just need something different. (Don't get so rule-oriented that color isn't fun anymore!)**

Personality

Some people like drama (really red, really gold, or really ash; really light or dark; unusual creative effects), but most people like it natural (muted colors—auburns or soft golds). Here we're talking about personality, or per-

Colorist's Clipboard

The level(s) and tone(s) most complimentary for a client depend on her:

- *Skin tone and eye color,*

- *Personality, and*

- *Haircut and style.*

Lili Jakel

color director at Michael Kluthe's Toronto, Ontario, salon:

"Suitability is everything . . .

a base that underscores what

she is and who she is, to add

dimension and softness, to

enhance skin and eye color. I go

"80 percent toward the skin . . .

"Trend is okay, but trend today

is unrealistic. How much effort,

time and maintenance is

involved? A more modern

blond is more realistic . . .

"Study your client, study your

product, and keep your

technique simple."

Gregory Carlyle

**owner of G. Carlyle Salon,
Winston Salem, North Carolina:**

"If you are going to create a

substantial change in someone,

you should always do the haircut

before the color. It is difficult

to think about what you can

do with the color unless you

get the cut in there first."

Colorist's Clipboard

**Communicating with the
color client:**

• *What change does she have
in mind—lighter, darker, a
different tone? What does
she want?*

• *What suits her natural coloring, especially her skin? Her
eyes? What will complement
her cut? Advise her.*

• *What can she afford?*

**Pinpoint the desired end
result in terms of level(s)
and tone(s).**

• *Write it down.*

sonal style. Is she casual, dramatic, or some-where in-between?

Haircoloring that suits who she is inside is the ideal. The purpose of hair is to beautify the wearer, and only she really knows what makes her *feel* beautiful. The section in this chapter entitled The Client's Preferences is really about personality. Personality is expressed in prefer-ences. People generally know what they can carry off, or will easily agree to it when shown. Because most people have an eye for color, clients rarely request colors that are genuinely unsuitable, and a client who has the wrong idea about her haircoloring will almost always accept the colorist's advice, if shown why.

There are lots of theories of personality (one of the best-known identifies people as natural, classic, dramatic, gamine, or roman-tic). Personality theories are fascinating, but not nearly as reliable as learning to conduct a good consultation—learning to listen and lead the client through an efficient, effective consultation.

The personality of a *color*, by the way—its individuality—is often in the details: the addi-tion of highlights; the placement, size, and color of highlights; the use of different colors to create dimension or shading; and how well you manipulate your color products to create certain tones and blends of tones.

Haircut and Style

Haircoloring should work hand-in-hand with the haircut. A good colorist always considers the cut. Color lends character to the form and affects the overall mood of the cut. "The form is the body of the color; the color is the soul of the form."[2] The compatibility of color and cut is subjective (subject to individual interpreta-tion and to swings in fashion) but to general-

ize, an avant-garde haircut calls for an avant-garde color; classic cut, classic color, and so on.

Moreover, color can and should be used to accentuate the form and details within it. Haircoloring is used to give texture and dimen-sion, or contour, to the cut. To an extent, hair-coloring can also contour the client's face.

Color contouring is based on **The Princi-ple of Light and Dark:**

**Light extends (maximizes);
Dark recedes (minimizes).**

Lighter, more luminous colors make areas appear more prominent, bringing the area for-ward or making it appear larger. So light color-ing can be used to create a focal point, to make hair look fuller, or to broaden a narrow face.

Dark colors make areas recede, or look smaller, closer, tighter. Depth, or shading, strengthens a weight line. Dark hair at the tem-ples slims a full face.

Combining light and dark creates texture and motion. Light next to dark makes the hair appear to have more movement and dimen-sion. Regarding dimensional haircoloring or other creative techniques, color should gener-ally be lighter where the cut is fuller and dark-er where the cut is shorter. Dark colors look more weighty and solid, whereas lighter colors look fuller and show more texture.

Variations in the overall coloring bring attention to that part of the design—what is different draws the eye. Lighter, darker, or tonally stronger coloring can be used to emphasize facial features or details in the cut—redder or blonder pieces in the bangs to accentuate the eyes, for instance.

---

2 Gerstner, K., The Forms of Color (Cambride, MA:
MIT Press, 1986).

Lili Jakel's Haircoloring Guide to Suit Your Skin and Eyes:

Very Pale Skin

Best Color Choices: Light golden, honey blond, reddish blond, golden auburn, light-to-deep golden brown, deep brunette.

Special Advice: Make skin warmer with golden haircoloring, avoid ashy and very pale blond shades.

Rosy Skin

Best Color Choices: Pale to ashy blonds, light-to-medium browns, muted auburns.

Special Advice: Tone down pink skin with ashy subdued haircoloring.

Sallow Skin

Best Color Choices: Golden blond, light-to-dark golden brown, deep rich brunettes.

Special Advice: Brighten olive or yellow skin with lighter, brighter haircoloring, no drab ash or pale blond shades.

Florid Skin

Best Color Choices: Sandy to ash blond, light-to-medium ash browns, muted auburns.

Special Advice: Tone down reddish skin with ash tones, avoid red colors.

Dark Skin

Best Color Choices: Soft auburn, deep reds, burgundy browns.

Special Advice: Black or dark skin may be sallow or have pink undertones. Nevertheless, hair color should stay dark. Only the tones should be changed to either warm goldens browns with auburn or cool burgundy browns, respectively.

The emphasis should be 80 percent on skin one, 20 percent on eyes. If you have made your decision depending on skin color, check the eye color and lean towards the following direction:

Blue Eyes—cooler tones

Blue-Green Eyes—sunny, lemon tones

Green Eyes—sunbronze, light red tones

Hazel Eyes—auburn, golden tones

Dark Eyes—cool or warm tones (depending on skin color)

The next time you pass by a competition room at a hair show, look at the coloring used. Color is used to perfection by the best competitors to enunciate the form with texture, movement, and detail.

RECAP

After analyzing the client's hair, begin defining with her exactly what you will accomplish today. Repeat back to her what you have heard her saying about her color. Ask the necessary questions to be certain you know what she wants. Show and tell her what her options are and what you think is best, in terms of level(s) and tone(s); write it down.

Before you settle on the service to be performed, though, there is one more matter to discuss: her time and money.

PRACTICALITY (THE MAINTENANCE FACTOR)

Can she afford it? How faithful about touch-ups will she be? The client needs to understand in advance the commitment she is making—

the late Jon Geunter

renowned colorist, founder of the Congress of Colorists (an organization of the 1970s), on communicating cost:

"Never disguise the cost of your professional haircoloring services. You and your client enter a business deal—the dollar amounts involved should be clear and correctly stated, which is good business no matter what business . . .

"Your client feels comfortable if she knows what her total bill will be. If it's a bit steep for her, she can lower the amount before you start. Like having only a partial highlighting, postponing her haircut, etc."

—*from* The Art of Blonding and Special Effects *(New York, NY: Clairol), p. 20.*

not that there are too many things in haircoloring that cannot be undone!

A four-week semi-permanent may be the best option, or a not-too-heavy highlighting or multishading, for the client who is wary of high maintenance. The more you change her natural color, the more maintenance it will require. Factor in the cost of any necessary treatments and a good shampoo and conditioner, too.

CONCLUSION

The best color choice for a client is a mix of what she subjectively prefers, what objectively suits her, and what is practical for her.

Greet your client, listen to her, evaluate her hair, listen some more, make recommendations, and get her go-ahead. Then you are prepared to formulate.

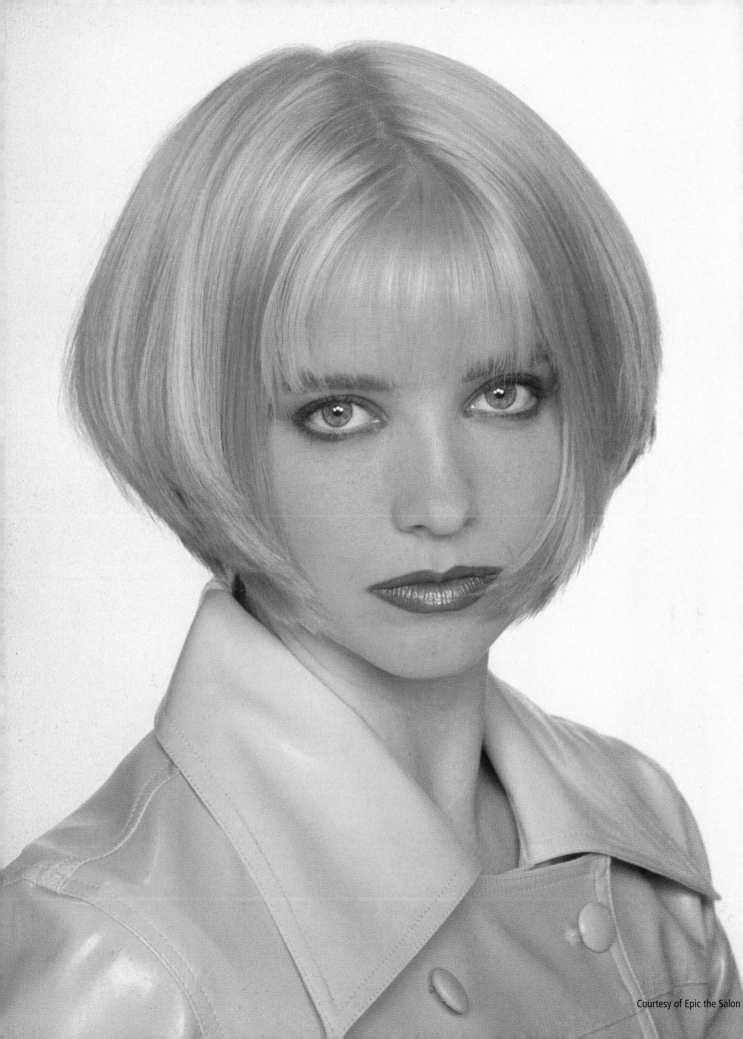

writing the formula

When the consultation is complete and you have settled on a desired end result, take your notes into the dispensary with you. That's where actual formulation occurs. Selecting the desired end result is not formulating; *formulating* is *deciding what will produce the desired end result*, based on the client's key factors: natural level, percentage of gray, texture, porosity (condition), and any existing haircoloring.

FORMULATION GUIDELINES

For specific information on color and developer selection, refer to your manufacturer's literature. The following guidelines are general rather than specific.

Developer Selection

Developer strength is dictated basically by how much lightening is required in the formula. Read your manufacturer's directions carefully in this regard. Higher volumes are used for higher lift. If you are not lifting, but are matching the natural base or going deeper, then standard usage (20 volume) is sufficient, and many companies tell you to use an even lower volume (10 or 15). To determine how many levels you are lifting, compare the client's natural base level to the target level. The difference between the two is the number of levels you are lifting.

Don't let this be a sticking point for you—it is extremely simple! Desired level minus natural level is the number of levels you are lifting. (DL – NL = Levels of Lift.) Count on your fingers if you have to (we all have!).

Generally speaking, up to 1 level of lift is achieved with 10 volume, up to 2 levels with 20 volume, up to 3 with 30, and up to 4 with 40. With most products, for instance, 20 volume would be used to go from a natural base of 5 to a target level of 7. To lift from a 5 to a 9, 40 volume would be required with most products.

There are certain products, (and there aren't very many of them) that use only 20 volume developer and so rely on higher levels of ammonia in the tint to create additional lift. These products use an "averaging" system of formula selection. Double the desired level and subtract the natural level to determine the level of tint to use when lifting.

Selecting the Level of the Formula

In most manufacturers' systems, the level you use is the level you get (as long as you do not exceed the lifting capability of the color). If you want to achieve a medium blond result, you use a medium blond formula; if you want to achieve a medium brown, you use a medium brown. You use your *target level,* in other words.

Variations on this rule do exist, however, so know your product.

On the one hand, you may be instructed to formulate *lighter* than the desired result unless the client is quite gray. On the other hand, if the client is very gray, you may be instructed to *deepen* your formula. These are exceptions, not the rule, but know your product!

One last, rare exception is the type of haircoloring system that uses only 20 volume developer. To achieve more than 2 levels of lift, you use lighter colors instead of higher developer volumes. When lifting, the level of the formula is determined by multiplying the desired level by two and subtracting the natural level. For example, a client who has a natural base of 4 and wants to be a 7 would be colored with a 10 level formula ($2 \times 7 = 14$, $14 - 4 = 10$), and 20 volume developer.

Selecting the Tone of the Formula

Now—the tone of the formula. This is what separates the experts from the beginners. And this is where really knowing your color line (the intensity of tones, the pigments in those tubes or bottles) comes in handy. If you are not yet familiar with the pigments in your system, including concentrates—also known as drops, drabbers, modifiers, mixers, intensifiers, fortifiers, mixtones, accents, kickers, creators, and jewel tones—then rely closely on the manufacturer's written recommendations.

If a client is unhappy with her haircoloring, it is almost always the tone she doesn't like. Have you noticed that? A client who comes into the salon with a color she hates, of your doing or someone else's, will almost always decry the *tone,* not the level. "Too brassy / Not red enough / Drab (too ash) / Don't I look orange to you?" This is where things can most easily go wrong, so apply yourself to getting it right.

The first step in getting the tone right is to be absolutely certain you know what your client needs and expects. The second step is to be sure you create that result, formulating with all her key factors in mind.

Natural base level tells you what kind of dominant underlying color the client has. In light of the desired end result, is that undertone a problem to be eliminated or an asset to be used? In other words, are you going to have to work to contrast-out her underlying color tone, or will it enhance the result?

Scenario 1: The client's natural base is a light brown, no gray, everything about her hair is normal. She wants to be a light neutral blond. What kind of undertone is characteristic of light brown hair? That's right—orange. You will be exposing and lifting tenacious red and gold pigment (lightening creates warmth). Ash is required to eliminate the unwanted warmth. Your formula, to achieve a neutral result, will consist of an ash-series color, probably with additional **drabber,** and a high-volume developer (meaning higher than the standard 20 volume).

Scenario 2: The same client wants to be a light golden blond. Now her natural underlying warmth is not such a liability, although it is still excessively warm. Depending on your color system, you will probably use a neutral series color to achieve a soft gold result—

remember you want to see gold, not orange; a little cool artificial pigment is probably in order (and by the way, most gold series are a tad cool, contradictory though that sounds).

Scenario 3: Let's say the same client wants to be a dark golden blond, a mere one level lighter. Lifting only one level, you will not be uncovering much natural warmth; to get a good golden result you would need to formulate with warmth—gold series and probably gold concentrate. (And using 20 volume will create more warmth than using a lower volume.)

Scenario 4: Now we have a new client, light brown but 50 percent gray. She wants to be a light neutral blond. What is the dominant underlying color of the 50 percent of her hair that is white? Trick question! White hair is essentially unpigmented, and ashy in appearance (ash is the absence of warmth). Use a true ash blond on this client and you won't get total coverage (depending on the product, you might even get an off-tone). So what do you do? You decide what is most important to the client—being light, and a completely neutral tone, or solid gray coverage. The lighter and cooler the formula, the sheerer the gray coverage will be. If she will accept a blend, without total coverage, then she can have her light neutral blond. Would you make this formula very drab? Of course not—there is 50 percent less warmth to contrast-out than in the first scenario we discussed, but it does have to be cool. A neutral formula, perhaps with some ash series in it, is a likely solution. If perfect gray coverage is what is most important to her, then she may need to accept a medium rather than a light blond, with some highlighting. (I have a client with a base of light brown, 40 to 70 percent gray, whom we bleach and tone to get both the flawless coverage and the light, absolutely neutral blond she

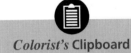

Colorist's **Clipboard**

Writing the formula:

- *Developer selection is based on how much you are lifting. Texture and condition should also be considered.*

- *The level of the formula usually corresponds to the desired, or target, level. (With some systems, percentage of gray changes the level you use. And with the systems that use no higher than 20 volume developer, lift is increased by using a higher-level tint instead of increasing the volume.)*

- *The tone of the formula depends on:*

  1. The desired tonal result,

  2. The dominant underlying color, and

  3. Porosity and texture.

wants—but most clients can be satisfied with single-process color.)

Scenario 5: Let's go back to that first client case, but change her texture. Light brown natural level, no gray, but coarse and glassy as horse hair, and she wants to be a light neutral blond. Better pull out all the stops! Boost up the developer, and ash it to the max! Depending on your color line, you might consider bleaching if she really wants an absolutely neutral result.

The theoretical formulas can go on forever, ad nauseam. Theoretical formulation is helpful, up to a point. The real secret to learning to formulate, though, is to formulate—to do color.

Formulating for Ethnic Hair

"What I try to impress upon my students," says John Sloan, owner of Chattanooga Beauty and

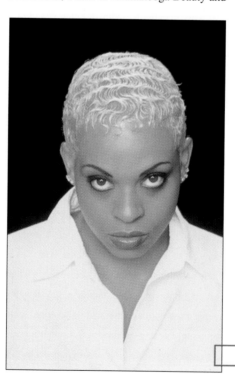

Courtesy of George Alderete for Sculpt Salon

Barber College, "is that African-American hair is subject to the same processes and you have to approach it the same way [as Caucasian hair]. You have to analyze the hair, and it depends on where you are starting from. Natural level may be 2 or it may be 5." (The enrollment at his school is 80 percent African-American, as is the clientele.)

The rules of formulation are the same for everyone; haircoloring doesn't know whose hair it is on. No matter what the client's ethnic background, the formula is based upon the key factors (natural level, percentage of gray, texture, porosity, and existing tint), the client's desires, what looks best on her, and what she can maintain.

If the hair has been subject to chemical relaxing, the condition (porosity) of the hair is of greater concern, though. Reginald Mitchell, Director of Training for a major manufacturer that specializes in products for African-American hair, says this: "On chemically treated hair, the first factor is the condition of the hair. The *second* factor is the natural color of the hair."

Using Professional Language

If you talk formulation within earshot of your client, use the professional language of numbers and letters, not color names. This is for her protection as well as yours. You are coloring her hair, not teaching her how to color her own hair. If she hears you say "light ash blond" she may think she can achieve the same result with the "light ash blond" on the drugstore shelf, and then she will have to pay to have it corrected.

The rules of formulation are the same for everyone; haircoloring doesn't know whose hair it is.

CONCLUSION

To do perfect haircoloring you must fully understand three things: the hair you are working with, your client's wishes, and your color line. Identifying the five key factors gives you what you need to know about the client's hair. Your client's wishes are discerned by active listening. Your color line is understood by reading all about it and then using it.

Read and know your manufacturer's literature; apply basic color principles; do a good, methodical analysis; communicate carefully with your client; and, when you mix, Keep It Simple, Sweetheart (KISS)! One other thing: every time you do a color, make sure you learn from it.

How Do You Know What Pigment Colors You Are Really Are Working With?

Manufacturers have various ways of conveying this information:

• Letters to indicate the dominant and secondary tones (BV = blue-violet dominant; OR = orange-red dominant, and so on). Uppercase letters for dominant tones; lower case for secondary tones (Rv = red dominant, violet secondary).

• Numbers to indicate dominant and secondary tones, or a combination of letters and numbers (.1 = ash, .3 = gold, and so on).

• Placement of each series on the color wheel (each tonal series positioned graphically on a color wheel).

• Placement on a continuum from coolest to warmest (tonal series positioned on a graph line from cool to warm).

• Percentages of primaries (content of each series expressed in percentages, for instance: 50 percent blue, 30 percent red, 20 percent yellow = natural series).

• Primaries expressed in "triads" (B for blue, R for red and Y for yellow). The same natural series represented above in percentages would be represented in triads as: BBBBBRRRYY.

• Verbal description ("Neutral base with added ash," "equal warm and cool pigments," "predominant base is blue," "neutral base with ash dominant," "predominant base is blue-green," "brown background with gold accent," and so on).

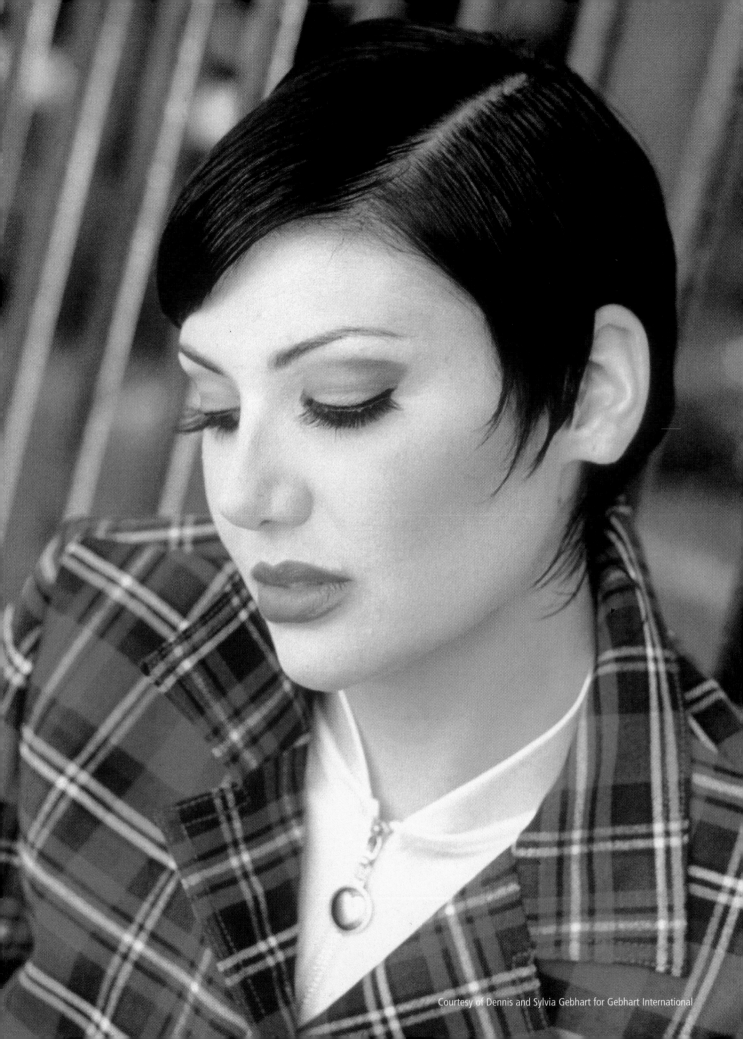

Courtesy of Dennis and Sylvia Gebhart for Gebhart International

the universal method of formulation— checklist and summary

The Universal Method of Formulation, based on universal color principles, is a general procedure for the planning and execution of salon color services. It is a systemized approach to color services that applies to all salon haircoloring—all brands and categories of products, and all types of color services.

CHECKLIST

1. **Analysis** (takes about one minute)
   - ❏ What is the client's natural base level?
   - ❏ Percentage of gray?
   - ❏ Texture?
   - ❏ Porosity?
   - ❏ Is there any existing tint on the hair?

2. **Communication** (takes another five minutes or so)
   - ❏ What end result does the client have in mind?
   - ❏ What range of levels and tones best suits her?
   - ❏ How much maintenance is she capable of?
   - ❏ Specifically, what color service do you recommend?

   Pinpoint the desired end result by level(s) and tone(s).

3. **Formulation**
   - ❏ A haircoloring result is the combined effect of the key factors and the formula used.
     Key Factors + Formula = Result
   - ❏ Given her key factors, what formula will produce the desired result?
   - ❏ Choose the appropriate:
     - ❏ Color(s)—level and tone
     - ❏ And developer (appropriate volume), per: manufacturer's directions. Measure and mix per: directions.

4. **Application**
   - ❏ Virgin application? Scalp to ends, or beginning ½" away from the scalp?
   - ❏ Retouch? How faded are the ends?
   - ❏ Select timing.

Andre Galuska

lifelong stylist, now at Saks Fifth Avenue, in Boca Raton, Florida, on formulation:

"I do color by eye. I don't use swatches, unless she asks to see them; I don't ask her what she's had before, what the hairdresser did before—all of that—forget it! I could care less. I ask two things: how much lighter (or deeper) she wants to be, and then [I assess] what she can afford. I look at her clothes, I ask her about her lifestyle, but only to decide what she can afford. Then I do the color by eye—I give her what she should wear."

SUMMARY

All haircoloring services consist of a consultation (analysis and communication), formulation, and application. Even if you don't plan it that way, that's how it will occur. You can't mix color before you have talked to your client; communication has to come before formulation. You can't fully advise your client about her options without knowing her key factors—analysis is first.

Whether it is semi-permanent, demi-permanent, permanent color, or bleach—virgin application, retouch, conversion to a different color product, corrective or creative color—haircoloring is always formulated in basically the same way. The same variables affect every haircoloring service, so the formulation procedure is always basically the same.

The variables that shape all color services are:

a. The five key factors (natural level, percentage of gray, texture, porosity, and existing tint),
b. The client's desires,
c. What looks best on her, and
d. What she can maintain.

Eventually, formulating becomes automatic. The method you practice becomes habit, second nature—automatic and almost subconscious.

Andre Galuska, source of the quote at left, has been a stylist for 37 years. For 22 years, he owned a successful salon in Westport, Connecticut. He did education for a major color company. When a color client sits in his chair, his eyes and hands instantly judge her hair, he talks briefly with her to establish what she wants and he recommends a color for her. This is what he calls, "doing color by eye." His kind of skillfulness is the product of experience and superb time management.

Ultimately, the Universal Method should be so second nature it becomes "color by eye." But "color by eye," that instant recognition of what the client needs and how to achieve it, is not a method that can be taught; it is the end result of experience.

The quickest way to develop expertise in haircoloring is to learn to think through formulation, that is what the Universal Method is—a thought process—rather than to learn rote formulas or to learn by trial and error. You do not have to have 37 years under your belt to do "color by eye;" you can develop expertise relatively quickly by making your experiences count.

The Consultation Process:

(Greeting)
• Listen to what she has
  in mind.

(Analysis)
• Identify the key factors; make notes.

(Communication)
• Repeat back to her what she has said she wants.

• Tell her what you recommend for her, and tell
  her the time and money involved.

• When you settle on the desired result, write it
  down.

(Formulation)
• Take your notes into the
  dispensary.

• Considering her key factors, what formula will
  produce the desired result?

How Much Time Does a Color Consultation Take?

For a client you know well, the complete color consultation will only take a few minutes. But for clients you don't know well, you will need more time—time to establish trust, as well as to establish what that person really wants and needs.

Even when a color client has been coming to you a long time you must never stop reevaluating her hair and offering her change. You don't ever want to take a client for granted or make her *feel* taken for granted.

Voula Fairbanks

co-owner of Hair Benders Internationale, Chattanooga, Tennessee:

"I don't spend more than three or four minutes on the consultation. More than that is not productive. If she can't make up her mind, I give her time to think about it—I walk away, do something else. A few minutes later I come back, put my hand on her shoulder and say, 'Are you ready to do this today?'—and I nod as I say it. 99 percent of the time she says yes and I send her back to get in a smock."

Jaime Escobedo

of Salon de Estee in Visalia, California:

"For a person that comes to me the first time for color [a new client getting color on the first visit] I like to spend at least twenty minutes on the consultation. I want to make sure that what they want is really the best for them—they're not just going through a divorce, or just lost a boyfriend!"

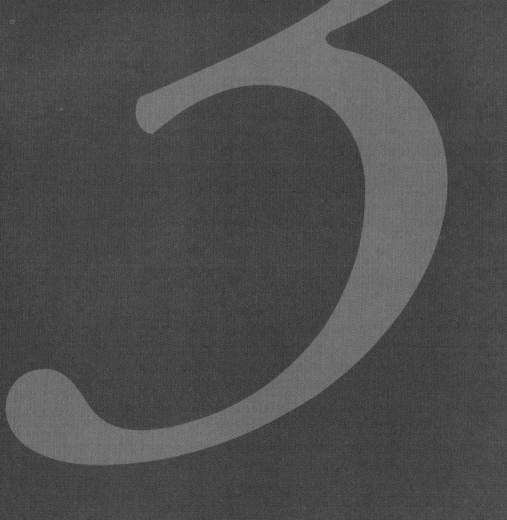

part three

the finer points of application and formulation

These next two chapters, Chapter Eight, Application Procedures, and Chapter Nine, Understanding the Main Service Categories (Gray Coverage, High-Lift Blonds, Reds, and Double-Process), elaborate on the basics of application and formulation.

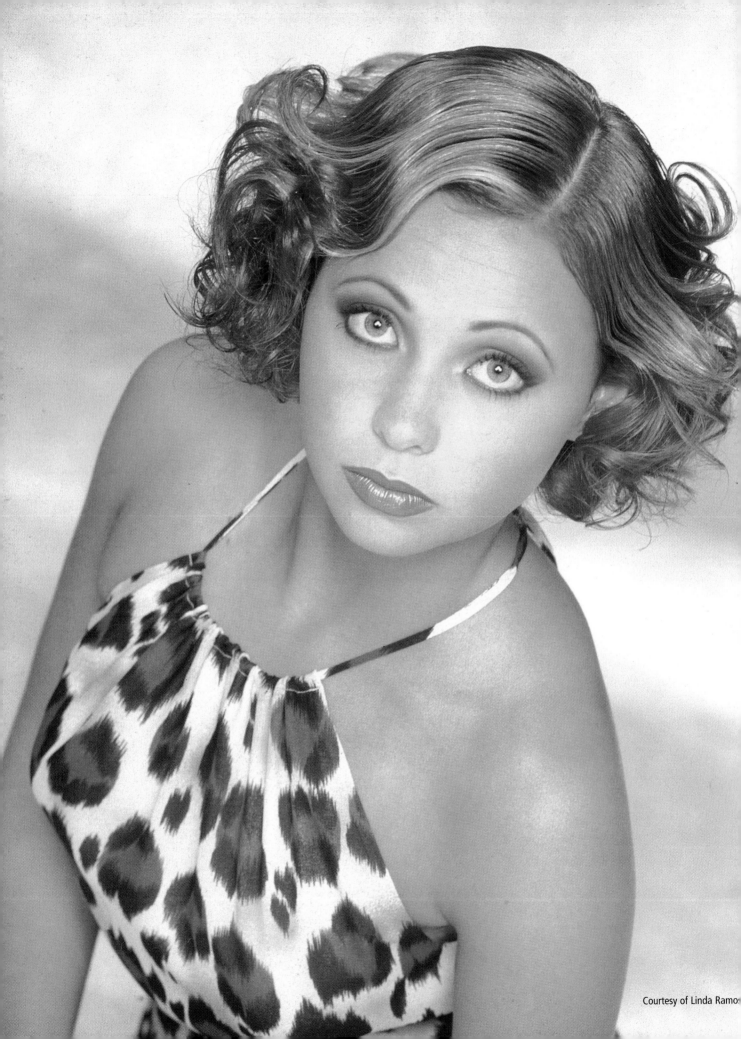

chapter eight

application procedures

Proper application and timing assure the success of a good formula. Good application cannot save a bad formula, but poor application can undermine the effort put into formulation. Errors in application and timing create as much corrective work as formulation errors.

Timing, something so simple, can make all the difference in the tone achieved, and in how well the haircoloring covers and wears. There is a proper way to rinse haircoloring, too. This chapter begins with two preliminary procedures: the patch test and the strand test.

PREDISPOSITION TESTING— ALLERGIES AND ALTERNATIVES

When you ask a new color client to relate her past haircoloring experiences, ask if she has ever experienced an allergic reaction or irritation with haircoloring. If a client has ever experienced discomfort that could be symptomatic of allergy (hives, redness, persistent itching, and so forth) do a predisposition test. Allergic reactions often worsen with subsequent exposure; the second reaction is usually worse than the first. An allergic client often knows what should and should not be used on her, and this is very helpful, but test to be certain that what you have planned will be safe.

Allergic Reactions and Finding Safe Alternatives

The component of haircoloring that is most **allergenic** is the dyestuff, and PPD (paraphenylenediamine) is the foremost—but certainly not the only—allergenic dye. All categories of haircoloring, and even bleaches, can induce allergic reactions. A client who is allergic to haircoloring will benefit from a trip to the dermatologist to determine which ingredients she should avoid; there may be safe alternatives.

Indicators of allergy include: swelling, irritation, redness, persistent itching or burning, rash, hives, blisters, broken or peeling skin, and anything else abnormal.

If a client is allergic to permanent haircoloring, or to any oxidation color (including demi-permanents), try patch testing a **nonoxidizing** semi-permanent (one which does not require a developing agent). True semi-permanents are frequently less offensive. Approximately three out of four people sensitized to permanent haircoloring can wear true semi-permanent haircoloring. (Remember, if the preparation of color involves mixing two parts together, it is not true semi-permanent haircoloring.) A pure henna product may be a good possibility as well, since henna is generally nonallergenic, and you might also consider a simple bleach highlighting.

It may be possible to use an **off-the-scalp technique** on an allergic client, but be oh-so-careful! Foils and frosting caps can bleed, and rinsing is a problem no matter what technique you use.

Incidence of allergy to oxidative haircoloring has been estimated at 1.3 of every 100 people. This means you can expect about 1 percent of your clientele to be allergic to permanent and demi-permanent haircoloring. This estimate probably represents the upper limit of incidence—improvements in haircoloring chemistry are continuously reducing the allergenicity of products and studies are often done on groups that are at greater risk for sensitivity—but you are guaranteed to eventually encounter allergic clients. Most reactions are mild, but some are quite severe. The most severe reactions occur with bleaches and involve respiratory problems; fortunately, these are much rarer than topical reactions from dyes. But don't underestimate the discomfort of hives and itching; remember, allergies only get worse.

And remember, too: if a client is allergic to permanent color, there is still a 75 percent chance that she can wear true semi-permanent haircoloring, and an excellent chance that henna will be safe.

The Importance of Wearing Gloves

For the stylist, excessive handling of dyes with bare hands may trigger sensitivity. The use of

You can expect about 1 percent of your clientele to be allergic to permanent and demi-permanent haircoloring.

gloves may help you to avoid **dye sensitization,** a potentially career-ending condition. Excellent, skinlike, powder-free gloves are now available and are a big improvement over the clumsy disposables.

How to Do a Predisposition Test

Instructions for **predisposition testing,** also called **sensitivity testing** or **patch testing,** are in every manufacturer's package insert and color manual; follow their directions. All companies teach almost exactly the same method.

Mix a small amount of the formula you plan to use. Always test the exact product and formula you intend to use on the client, with the intended developer. (There are different dyes in the different levels and tones of haircoloring; you want to test her sensitivity to the *exact* ingredients you are going to expose her to when you color her hair.)

Apply a dab of it to *clean* skin behind the client's ear or the inside of her elbow. It must remain there, undisturbed, for 24 hours. It may be necessary to loosely cover the formula with a Band-Aid so that the client doesn't absent-mindedly wipe it off or get it on her clothes. Make sure the bandage is somewhat loose, so that air can still reach the test area.

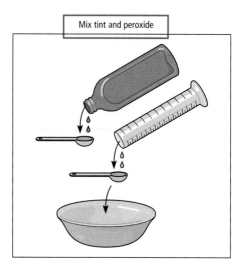

Mix tint and peroxide

After 24 hours, check your client's test area, watching for indicators of allergy: swelling, irritation, redness, persistent itching or burning, rash, hives, blisters, broken or peeling skin, and anything else abnormal.

PRELIMINARY STRAND TESTING

I once asked a stylist over the phone to do a preliminary **strand test.** She called me back 30 minutes later and told me she had done the strand test—applied the color all over the client's hair, then looked at a strand 15 minutes later! That was a classic communication failure; I obviously had not adequately explained what I meant her to do.

Strand testing is normally done *before* color goes on all over, in order to evaluate how well a given formula will work. If it doesn't work perfectly, you then have a chance to adjust it, based on what the hair has shown you. That is the purpose of strand testing: to evaluate a given formula, and make any necessary adjustments to it, before you do the complete application.

Sometimes you look at a strand of hair while an application is processing, to see how the color is developing or to see if it is ready to be rinsed, but this is not usually what is meant by the term *strand test.* It usually means a preliminary strand test—a preview of coming attractions!

How to Strand Test

When you test, test the exact formula you plan to use. You will be mixing a very small quantity of color, so be exacting about ratios—of color to color, if you are using more than one color, and of color to developer.

Apply the test formula to enough hair to really see the result—a square half-inch or

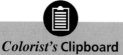

Colorist's **Clipboard**

Predisposition testing:

• *A client who is allergic to permanent or demi-permanent haircoloring may be able to wear semi-permanent haircoloring or henna.*

inch, depending on density—either from scalp to ends or in the most questionable area. If you are strand testing because of overporosity, test the most overporous hair on the client's head. If it is gray coverage that concerns you, test where the hair is grayest. If lightening, test where the hair is darkest.

Time the test strand normally for normal hair; overporous hair will process more quickly.

When you are ready to view the result, get all the color off the strand, and get it dry, before you judge it. (Lay the strand on a clean towel. Spritz it with water, wipe it, spritz it, wipe it, until the hair is clean. Then, rub the test strand dry, or dry it with a blower, and hold it against a clean white towel.) Then you can really see what the test formula did.

Strand Testing the Length while the Regrowth Processes

This is the most-used form of strand testing. When retouching a client with overporous length, you can easily strand test the length while the regrowth processes. If the scalp area is normal, but you aren't sure about the length, go ahead and get the formula on the regrowth, then apply to only a strand of the overporous length. Within five to ten minutes you should be able to see if and how much you will have to adjust the formula for the length. This is a time-saver; the overporous hair will take much less processing time than the scalp area, so you have time to work out the formula for the ends.

MEASURING AND MIXING

Developer ratios are very important. Measure both color and developer every time you mix—don't guess. Color-to-developer is a rather delicate balance. Refer to product inserts for specific guidelines, and adhere to them. All color tubes have increment markings; beakers, cups, or bottles are used to accurately measure liquid color or developer. If you must measure a small quantity of color, it will usually be measured in inches, capfuls, or metrically in centimeters or cubic centimeters (cc's), and most color bowls have unit markings on the bottom.

When you mix, mix thoroughly. Tube colors blend better if you stir the color cream or gel before adding the developer, and if you add the developer gradually rather than all at once. **Color shakers** are terrific for mixing color quickly and thoroughly (a shaker is a color bowl with a lid). I have also known salons to whisk hard-to-mix cream colors with a plastic fork, or a miniature stainless steel whisk.

Shortly after tint is mixed, it begins oxidizing, and oxidized tint can't color the hair. Don't mix until you are ready to apply. If an application takes much longer than 15 or 20 minutes, as in the case of a full head of foils, it is usually best to mix fresh color. Mix in small quantities, as needed. Keep the developer in a measuring cup, and the color in a bowl or bottle, at your station.

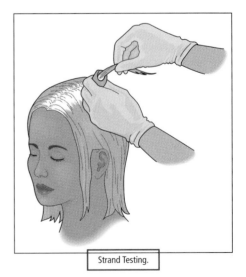

Strand Testing.

APPLICATION

There are two basic types of application: **virgin** and **retouch**.

Virgin Application of Permanent Haircoloring

A virgin application is first-time color—haircoloring on hair not previously color-treated.

For permanent haircoloring, there are two types of virgin application: **scalp-to-ends** and **double-application.** The nature of the color service determines which is appropriate.

Scalp-to-ends virgin application. For formulas the same level as, or darker than, the client's natural base, the method of virgin application is scalp-to-ends—*except for reds.* The reds of permanent haircoloring are not applied scalp-to-ends. If you are matching the client's natural base, or going darker than her base, and you aren't making her red, then you may simply apply the color scalp-to-ends.

Double-application method of virgin application. For formulas lighter than the natural base level and for bright formulas (reds and strong golds), application is begun ½″ away from the scalp. The scalp area lifts faster, so you stay away from it to start with; the midshaft and ends are given a head start. Application is begun ½″ away from the scalp and allowed to process briefly before fresh color is applied to the scalp area. The lighter or brighter the formula, the more important it is to use this double-application method. Because most clients go lighter or go red, this is usually how virgin color is applied.

The details of virgin application are just a little different with different products, so read your manufacturer's literature well. Generally speaking, when the double-application method

is used, the timing of that first application, begun ½″ away from the scalp, will be about half the full timing of the product. Then a *fresh* batch of color is mixed and applied to the scalp area. You may be instructed to wipe off the first application and apply the second batch scalp-to-ends (coloring the midshaft and ends twice), or to apply it only to the scalp area. In any case, the second application is given full processing time.

This method is used for lightening and reds because it is easier to make the scalp area light or bright than it is to lighten and brighten the length. If applied scalp-to-ends, red tint will appear brighter at the scalp area, and high-lift tint will lighten more at the scalp and appear deeper and warmer on the length. To achieve even lightening, color is first applied to the hair that will take the longest: the midshaft and ends.

For example: a client with a natural base of medium brown, normal porosity, is tinted a medium golden brown or a medium ash brown. For either, a scalp-to-ends application is fine. But if she were going red-brown or red, then the application would need to be begun ½″ away from the scalp, in order to achieve an even result. Were she going much lighter than her natural base level, the application would again be started ½″ away from the scalp.

You've seen home bleach jobs—scalp area nearly white and length, raw gold. Applied scalp-to-ends, high-lift tint also lightens more at the scalp. And how many times have you seen a gorgeous red with a dismayingly bright scalp? Improper application can create or contribute to these undesirable effects, and nothing looks more amateurish. (Don't let such results walk out of the salon uncorrected!)

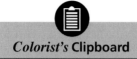

Colorist's Clipboard

Measuring and mixing

- Measure both color and developer.

- Mix just before applying.

- Mix thoroughly.

- Mix fresh color if an application with permanent haircoloring takes more than 20 minutes, as in the case of foils.

Dr. David Cannell

Senior V.P. of Research and Development for a major color manufacturer, conducted a study on why hair close to the scalp lightens faster. Is it due to body heat, or is it because the hair closest to the scalp isn't as hard? He concluded that body heat is the more important factor:

"Average room temperature is considered to be about 70°F; the temperature of the human body is 98.6°F or 37°C, and a warm hair dryer is 110°F. Body temperature is almost the equivalent of a warm dryer. You can imagine why, then, you get that banding effect with high-lift blonds and hot roots with reds that are applied scalp-to-ends. When we color swatches in the lab we process them at [98.6°F or] 37°C, not at room temperature . . . Cosmetologists also make use of body heat to process perms, trapping heat with plastic caps."

There are two theories about why the scalp area lifts more easily.

1. **The hair closest to the scalp is not as fully keratinized, or hardened, as the length. The newly keratinized new growth is softer and more amenable to lightening.**
2. **The warmth of the scalp increases lightening. The first quarter-inch or so surrounding the scalp is called the warm zone; it has the benefit of body heat (the mid-shaft is called the cold zone). Heat accelerates coloring, especially lightening.**

Overporous Ends

A virgin application on multiporous hair is a little different. Very overporous ends are left out of the application initially. With the double-application method, the color is first applied only to the midshaft, starting ½″ away from the scalp, up to the area of overporosity—both the warm zone (the scalp area) and overporous ends are left out to begin with. While the midshaft begins to process you strand test the ends to determine the necessary timing. Usually, overporous ends will process about as fast as the warm zone; when you go back and put color on the scalp area, you apply to the ends, also.

Virgin Application of Semi-Permanent Haircoloring

True semi-permanent color does not lighten natural pigment, so the method of virgin application is simply scalp-to-ends. However, bright or deep semi-permanent colors will stain the scalp, and are therefore applied just barely off-scalp. In addition, overporous ends will take on more tone or depth (with a red

semi-permanent, for example, overporous ends will be redder), so application and timing may be adjusted to get an even result on multi-porous hair.

Retouch Application

Retouches are self-explanatory, for the most part: Apply the formula to the regrowth, avoid overlapping, and pull it through as needed. But retouches are not entirely routine. How you proceed varies with the formula, the desired result, and with the quality of the hair on which you are working.

Timing on the length is determined basically by how much fadage has occurred. Many clients need color on their length with every retouch, but some do not. Sometimes all you need to color is the new growth. A client who desires translucency may do better without repeated application to her length. In certain cases, it can be detrimental to repeatedly pull color through. With a very drab, high-lift formula, for instance, pulling color through every time could easily result in off-color ends.

When retouching multiporous hair, timing on the overporous length may be very brief. Some colorists dilute the leftover color with an equal amount of water, or dampen the length, before pulling it through. You might also do what used to be called a **soapcap**, which doesn't involve soap at all; it means emulsifying the color through at the shampoo bowl—wetting the hair and working the wet color into a lather for a minute or two before rinsing.

On very overporous hair, an entirely different formula may be the best approach. Have you ever had a high-lift client whose ends became almost colorless? What you use to lift her new growth is not appropriate for her ends. To restore tone and depth to her ends, an entirely different formula is required: low-volume and warm.

Semi- or demi-permanent coloring may be used to refresh the length as well (permanent color on the new growth, and a corresponding semi- or demi-permanent on the ends). This is often kinder to the hair and more satisfactory tonally, and clients will love you for it.

When Is a Retouch Not a Retouch?

When the client has waited too long! Then it becomes a virgin application again, of sorts.

Let's say you have a client whom you lift four levels. She slips up and doesn't get into the salon for ten or twelve weeks. Now she has a 1½″ outgrowth. This is no longer a normal retouch.

If you were to simply apply her formula to that entire 1½″ regrowth, processing it as though it were a normal regrowth, she would be banded. The hair closest to her scalp would lift as expected, but a half-inch away from her scalp she would be less light and well-toned. In a case like this, the retouch should be treated as a virgin application. You would first apply the formula ½″ away from her scalp, up to her line of demarcation. Process that per manufacturer's directions, then apply to the warm zone.

Application of Color to Damp versus Dry Hair

Preshampooing is often advisable with the less penetrating, deposit-only products (demi- and semi-permanents). Hairspray or styling products are more of an impediment to these less aggressive colors, and some moisture in the hair helps even out the highs and lows of porosity when you are using the more porosity-sensitive products. Permanent haircoloring, though, is still generally applied to dry hair. There is rarely any reason, technically, to preshampoo before permanent color—permanent haircoloring will go right through whatever cosmetic film is on the hair—but some colorists just like to apply to clean, damp hair and, if it is properly done, there is no reason, technically, not to preshampoo.

If you preshampoo, go easy on the scalp. Think of how you brush a client before color; you brush the hair, not the scalp. Preshampooing is light and gentle, just enough to clean the hair. Towel the hair well before application and apply to damp rather than wet hair; you want the hair manageably moist, not dripping.

You may prefer application on dry hair, or you may find application to damp hair to be easier and quicker. It depends on your product, technique, and preference.

(Note: If there is a residue of heavy moisturizers or oils on the hair, such as those used to maintain ethnic hair, shampoo the hair thoroughly prior to coloring. Excessive oil lessens the deposit and lastability of any haircoloring. Semi-permanent color generally can't be maintained with oily after-care products.)

General Tips Regarding Application

1. **Haircoloring should be applied methodically. Quarter the hair: part her center front to center back, and ear to ear, then apply along these part lines first.**
   Or apply in a circular pattern, beginning at the crown. Whatever your method, if you apply color the same way every time you will work more quickly and are less likely to miss spots.
2. **Taking thin sections is actually faster than taking fewer but thicker (and harder-to-saturate)**

Preshampooing is light and gentle, just enough to clean the hair.

sections. The color will go on more evenly, too.

3. Color is always applied first to any area that will require the longest timing—the grayest area when covering gray, the darkest area when lightening.

4. A good application saturates the hair thoroughly, but does not smother it. Oxidation color needs exposure to oxygen. Don't be stingy—wet the hair thoroughly, envelope it thinly in color—but don't cake it on. Don't pack the hair together for processing, either. Loosen the hair; separate the strands, so that air can get to it. (True semi-permanent color and bleach are different; you won't choke them off by laying the hair together. Bleach does better, in fact, when the strands are laid together.)

5. When your application is complete, check it. Always check, even if you think it's perfect. Fugi Escobedo, salon owner, color master, and owner of a fine school in Atlanta, Georgia, once told me that "just when you think you have it perfect is probably when you don't!"

THE IMPORTANCE OF PROPER TIMING

Unless the manufacturer states otherwise, timing is begun when the application is complete. Lay the brush or bottle down and pick up the timer.

All products have a minimum and a maximum timing. It is almost never advisable to deny a formula the product's minimum timing.

If the manufacturer says the timing of the product is 30 to 45 minutes, every color should be allowed at least 30 minutes at the new growth. When maximum lift and deposit is desired, the product's maximum timing should be used. With most color products, frankly, most applications should be allowed the maximum timing.

High-lift colors should generally be allowed maximum timing, in order to tone the natural warmth that lightening creates (and to keep it toned until her next retouch). With gray coverage, the whole point is deposit; if she wants it covered and to stay covered, maximum timing should be used. And if any color is going to fade, it will be reds; to minimize fadage, the maximum timing is used. Any client that tends to fade should be allowed the maximum timing.

Gray coverage, high-lift, reds, and anyone who fades—what's left? Not much. There are some clients who do perfectly well with the minimum timing, such as clients with very fine hair, a gray client that wants only a blend, or a client whom you are lifting just a level or two, but these are the minority.

A few permanent haircoloring products have a different approach to timing; they prescribe timing based on the developer volume used—the higher the volume, the longer you leave the color on. The minimum timing might be 20 minutes, using 10 volume hydrogen peroxide; with every 10 volume increase in developer strength you increase timing by another ten minutes (30 minutes for 20 volume, 40 minutes for 30 volume, and so on).

On a retouch, the timing you give the length depends on how much the hair has faded, and it isn't always necessary to pull color through. If you aren't sure, strand test. Timing on overporous ends can be very, very brief.

Color Processing Machines (Lights and Steamers)

Timing is shorter when **infrared lights** or **steamers** (oxidizer, mist, or ozone machines) are used. Processing time is about one-third to one-fifth the normal timing; a 30-minute process takes about six to ten minutes; a 45-minute process takes nine to fifteen minutes. The recommended method of application may be different as well.

Not many color companies advocate the use of lights or steamers, but ask colorists who use them and you'll get resounding endorsements. Clients almost always appreciate the faster processing, too.

THE IMPORTANCE OF PROPER RINSING

If you have any uncertainty at all about the readiness of a color, check to see that you've got what you want before you rinse. Checking before rinsing can save having to reapply.

To check a color result, wipe the tint off a strand about as thick as a finger. Lay the strand on a towel, spritz the strand with water, wipe it, spritz it, wipe it, until it is clean. Then rub it with a clean towel until dry, or dry it with a blower, and place it against a clean, white towel—then you can see what you've got.

Proper Rinsing

The first order of business at the shampoo bowl is the removal of skin stains. Don't wet the hairline—wetting the hairline before lifting the stains will set them into the skin—but emulsify the haircoloring with a sprinkle of water and work it into a lather. With permanent or demi-permanent color use the hair around the face as an abrasive to eliminate the stains; rub the hair around the hairline vigorously into

any color on the skin. Using your gloved hand, work the hair, dye still on it, into the stains. You may feel like you are making more of a mess, but you aren't. Wipe the hairline to see if you have eliminated the stains; if not, go at it again, using the color itself and the hair as an abrasive. Remove any remaining shadow with **skin stain remover.** If you run out of skin stain remover, rubbing alcohol does pretty well. (Should you encounter a client whose skin really retains dye stains, note it on her client record and, in the future, apply a protective cream to her skin prior to application.)

Now—rinse! rinse! rinse! Always rinse haircoloring thoroughly before shampooing. If shampoo goes into the hair before the haircoloring is rinsed out, you begin fading the color that very moment (the shampoo goes into the hair where the new color molecules are and begins pulling them out), so rinse until the water runs clear, and *then* shampoo. Her hair will be so clean when you are done rinsing that she won't appear to need shampoo, but shampoo, to eliminate any unseen residue, and to halt the action of the haircoloring chemicals.

Water and shampoo begin restoring the hair back to an acid pH. Most manufacturers specifically recommend following-up with an **acid rinse,** to smooth the hair and to neutralize any trace of alkalinity that might remain in it. This is good general practice with any oxidation tint. When H_2O_2 is not fully eliminated from the hair, **creeping oxidation** can occur, further lightening the hair, and weakening it, too.

Wet Hair Does Not Show True Color

Clients frequently ask how their color looks while their hair is being rinsed. Reassure the client, *but do not judge color wet.* If she presses you for specifics, tell her you can't tell with her

Colorist's Clipboard

Proper timing:

• *Use a timer.*

• *Leave the color on the prescribed timing for that type of formula.*

• *Maximum timing gives you maximum lift and deposit.*

• *Color machines (lights and steamers) accelerate processing.*

• *If you aren't sure that the color is ready, check it before you rinse.*

hair wet. Remind clients who head straight for a mirror that wet hair does not show true color. (Mirrors are not helpful in the shampoo area!)

Some color mishaps can be caught and corrected right at the shampoo bowl, but this is a skill which is more learned than taught. It takes experience to know what you are really seeing. All color looks different when it is wet, and the specific product, the porosity of the hair, and the color tone all influence how haircoloring looks when it is wet. It also takes experience to know which products and procedures quickly eliminate minor problems. So don't jump to apply additional color on a still-wet head. Dry the hair, or at least a fistful of hair, then evaluate the success of the color service.

Semi-temporary and semi-permanent products (pigmented shampoos and conditioners, color-and-shine glazes, or other semi-products) are commonly used to correct minor tonal problems at the shampoo bowl. A demi-permanent product might be a good choice to deepen, to cover missed gray, or to blot spots where your bleach foils bled. You might use a high-lift tint to gently lighten ends that went too deep. (You will find more information on corrective techniques like these in Part Four: Corrective Haircoloring.)

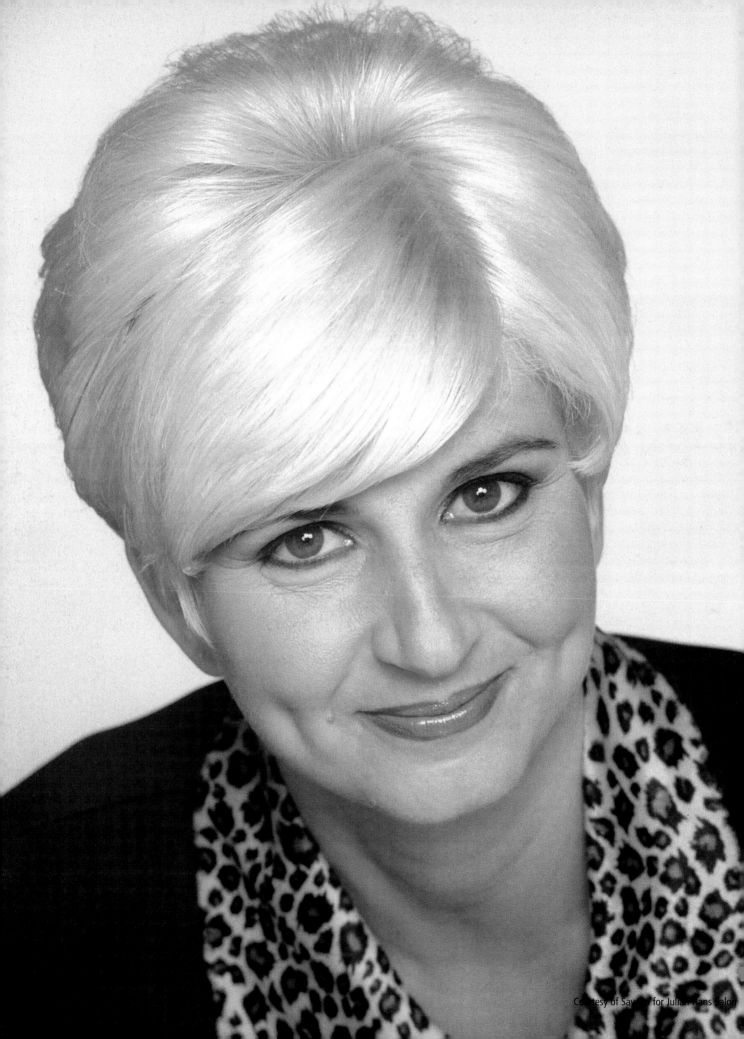

understanding the main service categories (gray coverage, high-lift blonds, reds, and double-process)

G ray coverage, high-lift blonds, and reds together comprise the bulk of salon haircoloring. These are the three main types of color changes that clients undergo. There are distinctly different considerations when it comes to formulating for deposit on gray versus high-lift or reds. And double-process— the use of scalp bleach—is a specialty in itself.

Much of the information in this unit is actually presented in preceding chapters, at intervals and often in the form of examples. This recap is provided due to the overriding importance of the material, and to supply a quick reference on each of the four subjects.

UNDERSTANDING GRAY COVERAGE

There are people who look good with a lot of gray, or with 100 percent gray—but not many. Let's face it: gray hair ages people. It almost always dulls the appearance. As much of a problem as those gray hairs are, the still pigmented hair loses shine and intensity as the person ages, too. Just as makeup improves almost any woman's appearance, so does coloring the gray. No woman or man wants to appear older than necessary. People who look older *feel older,* and people like to feel young.

The words *gray* and *white,* though technically different, are used interchangeably in this book. The difference between the two is one of degree, the degree to which the hair strands are unpigmented. A white strand contains no pigment, a gray strand contains minimal pigment. For purposes of haircoloring, however, gray and white hair are the same. It is *percentage* of gray that makes the difference in formulation. Percentage of gray is one of the key factors and should be estimated in advance of formulation.

Formulating to Cover Gray

Understanding what gray hair is, or what it is not, explains much about the way it accepts haircoloring. Gray hair is basically unpigmented, and this is primarily what makes formulation different. In addition, gray hair is often resistant.

Gray hair, lacking pigment, lacks both the depth and the underlying warmth of pigmented hair. To cover gray, you must replace what is missing from it. Gray hair lacks warmth. Consequently, warm formulas cover better than cool formulas. Gray hair also lacks depth, and with some—but not all—products, formulas will look substantially lighter on gray hair than they do on pigmented hair.

When you use warm haircoloring on gray hair, you are in effect replacing missing underlying warmth; tint supplies what the pigment-producing cells of the hair no longer do. It is primarily gold artificial pigment that accomplishes coverage. Just slight warmth makes a huge difference in how the formula covers—neutral colors contain some warm dyes and give markedly better coverage than ash colors.

Before you can deposit the dyes that cover the gray, though, you have to get past the resistant outer layer typical of gray hair. Very low developer volumes (below 10 volume) are insufficient to soften and penetrate resistant hair. With most products, 15 to 20 volume is ideal for coverage. High volumes—higher than the standard 20 volume—will soften the cuticle, but they also decrease deposit and lessen the coverage.

Selecting the Desired Level

Be wary of tinting a graying client too dark. Although she may *think* she wants to be the color she once was, it may be a mistake. She may not wear depth as well as she once did and,

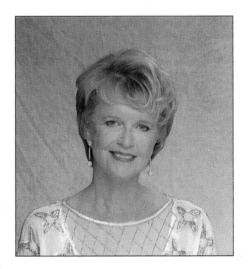

> Gray hair, lacking pigment, lacks both the depth and the underlying warmth of pigmented hair.

in any case, she is accustomed to being gray, which is lighter. Here's a rule of thumb: if under 50 percent gray, go one level lighter than the natural base; if over 50 percent gray, two levels lighter. Clients who want a natural-looking result often do better with a technique or formula that blends, rather than covers, their gray.

Dark colors can look severe, as you know, but so can ultralight colors. In general, extremes tend to become less complimentary with age.

Ash Formulas on Gray Hair

Gray hair is, by its very nature, ash, as ash is the absence of warmth. Therefore, ash artificial pigment alone does not cover gray. It does not supply what gray hair lacks. Ash on gray, which *is* ash, looks very ash indeed, and blends rather than covers. The higher the percentage of gray, the less ash covers.

Depending on the nature and intensity of its artificial ash pigment, ash haircoloring on gray hair may produce off-tones. Manufacturers are quite clear about whether or not their ash colors can be used on gray hair. Some ash haircoloring is perfectly okay to use on gray hair, usually, however, with the addition of a neutral (natural) color, and without the expectation of total coverage. Other ash products will create blue, green, or violet tones. Artificial ash pigment is specifically designed to offset natural warmth, and there is none—or almost none—in gray hair.

Red Formulation on Gray Hair

Because gray hair lacks depth, red haircoloring appears brighter on it. Imagine a red marker on white paper versus the same red marker on brown paper. Red paint on a white canvas versus red paint on a brown canvas; which appears brighter?

Whereas a red-brown series is probably acceptable, vibrant reds will appear unacceptably garish on high percentages of gray.

In order for red haircoloring to produce vibrant results on pigmented hair, the dyes have to be very, very brilliant indeed. Gray hair does not have any natural depth to mute bright red artificial pigment. On someone with a high percentage of gray, an intense red will look like a clown's wig. A bright red formula on bleached hair would yield a similarly garish result. The very strongest reds are designed with pigmented hair in mind.

To produce bright but believable reds on gray hair, the formula is generally muted with a less-bright color of the same level (a red-brown, red-blond, or a golden or neutral brown or blond). The formula is made less bright, because red tint on gray hair appears more bright.

Blond Formulas on Gray Hair

Very light colors do not cover gray as well as light to medium blonds, and deeper. Blonds lighter than a light blond are really meant to lift natural pigment, not cover gray. Pale blonds have more lift than deposit, which is counter to coverage of gray; gray coverage is all about maximizing deposit, not lift. Pale blonds just don't have the pigment necessary to replace missing depth and really provide coverage. Such colors can be used for blending gray, though: the paler the blond the more sheer the blend.

Lifting more than two levels above natural base tends to lessen coverage, because using higher than the standard 20 volume developer means sacrificing some deposit for lift. For clients who want to be blond, this is an acceptable trade-off. Almost without exception, being light is more important to the client than

Dark colors can look severe, but so can ultralight colors.

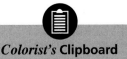

perfect coverage. A client with a natural base of dark brown and 50 percent gray, for example, will not usually get perfect coverage if she is colored dark to medium blond (using 30 or 40 volume), but if you achieve the right level and tone, she will gladly accept a blend.

Imagine you have a 50 percent gray, dark brown client who wants to be dark to medium neutral blond. If you were to bleach and tone, you could get perfect coverage and any tone you wanted. Using single-process haircoloring, though, you have to formulate more to eliminate natural underlying warmth than to cover gray. That means using cool tones and a high-volume developer, which will give you less coverage.

Remember that warmth covers gray better than does ash. The missing underlying pigment that must be replaced when you cover gray is gold. Golden blonds cover gray best. The addition of gold concentrate is often required to cover or achieve golden tones on high percentages of gray. Depending on the system, most gold series colors will look neutral to just barely golden (some even look ash) on an 80 to 100 percent gray head of hair.

Developer Selection for Gray Coverage

The key to choosing the right developer for gray coverage is to select the lowest volume capable of softening the cuticle, usually 15 to 20 volume. Typical gray hair has a wiry texture, a tough, compact cuticle. The more resistant the gray, and the coarser the gray, the harder it is to penetrate—too weak a developer won't soften it. And when maximum deposit is the imperative, high volumes should be avoided, as well. Higher than the standard 20 volume, in most systems, will reduce deposit.

APPLICATION AND TIMING FOR GRAY COVERAGE

Application for gray coverage is begun where the client is grayest.

Coarse, resistant gray can be tricky to fully saturate. Wiry gray hairs can separate themselves from the rest of the application (like they spring out of a perm rod) and tend to dry out, especially around the hairline. Good gray coverage requires a heavy application. Double-check your application, as always.

Don't be stingy with the color: *Really soak it, but don't choke it!* Oxidation tint should not be so heavily applied that air can't get to it.

With many products, the best method of virgin application for gray coverage is the double-application method for first-time color. The first time her hair is colored, begin by applying ½ inch away from the scalp, out to the porous ends; wait 15 or 20 minutes, blot the excess tint from the hair and, using fresh color, apply scalp-to-ends. This is similar to presoftening or prepigmenting (you are coloring the hair twice).

Maximum timing assures maximum deposit, and gives the best coverage of gray. Proper timing is of great importance to good, lasting coverage. When you do retouches, allow the maximum timing on the regrowth. Timing on the ends depends on how much fadage has occurred.

Blending versus Coverage of Gray

Some clients want every strand covered, and they want it to stay that way until their retouch. But it is not always total coverage that best suits a gray or graying client. Some people like to keep a few "executive highlights"—a little silver spun in the gold. Men, especially, often want to avoid such an obvious change that everyone will be remarking about it at work the next day. A blend, rather than coverage, often suits them best.

A blend has dimension and shimmer, and this is very natural-looking. A **blend** means lots of strands covered, lots just toned, and a few still white. The haircoloring product, as well as the tone, depth, developer, application, and timing of the formula, can be selected to achieve a blend rather than coverage.

Some color products are specifically designed to blend rather than cover gray. Semi-permanent products blend, and some blend only very low percentages; demi-permanents may either blend or cover; permanent products cover, some more solidly than others. And any haircoloring product can be manipulated to minimize rather than maximize coverage.

When a client desires only a blend, color may be applied less solidly, particularly around the face. Use a comb to lightly apply the formula; do not saturate every strand, leave some untouched. This gives a very natural appearance, especially for men, and avoids any obvious outgrowth. **Highlighting** or **lowlighting** are also options for the client who doesn't want complete coverage.

Semi- and demi-permanent haircoloring can be very effective for blending gray, but not always. There are clients whose gray is so tenacious that it is completely unaffected by semi-permanent and even demi-permanent haircoloring. Some gray hair simply requires the penetration of permanent haircoloring.

Brightening Gray Hair

Even if a client wishes to keep her gray, most gray hair will yellow from cigarette smoke, sun, perming, and hard water, and really should be treated with a semi- or demi-perma-

nent product to keep it ash (snowy, silvery, smoky, or steely). If a haircoloring product can be used for this purpose, the manufacturer will specifically say so.

If You Have Trouble Getting Coverage

If you are having trouble getting total gray coverage, reread your manufacturer's literature thoroughly. First be sure you are using the tones, depth, developer, and timing recommended for coverage. If you are, and you are still not getting complete coverage, the literature may recommend presoftening, prestaining, prepigmentation, double pigmentation, or some other such technique. Don't hesitate to call the manufacturer's toll-free phone number for help.

UNDERSTANDING HIGH-LIFT BLONDS

There are two sides to the high-lift story—lightening natural pigment, and toning remaining natural warmth—both occurring, of course, in a single process.

Lift

Permanent haircoloring can only lift so much, usually four levels. Some products achieve five levels of lift with the use of a special high-lift series or with the addition of a booster. Beyond that, the client becomes a candidate for double-process (prelightening).

The lifting capability of a formula has two origins: the volume strength of the developer and the amount of ammonia in the dye-bearing liquid, gel, or cream. The lighter (higher) the level of tint, the more ammonia it contains and the greater its potential lifting capability. The higher the volume of developer, the greater the lift. Anything stronger than 20

A blend means lots of strands covered, lots just toned, and a few still white.

volume is considered high-lift hydrogen peroxide. Manufacturers' directions must be followed to a "T" regarding developer selection and color-to-developer ratio in order to achieve the best lightening.

Every system tells you not to exceed a certain number of levels of lift, and most tell you to use the level formula you wish to achieve.[1] To defy the directions is an exercise in futility. You can't wish the product into doing more than it is designed to do.

Toning

Lightening creates warmth; when natural pigment is lightened, the natural underlying warmth of the hair is exposed. If a warm result is undesirable, then *ash* artificial pigment must be used to contrast-out the unwanted warmth. (Lightened natural pigment + artificial pigment = the color result.)

The more you lift, the more warmth you create, and the ashier the formula must be to avoid a warm result.

Not every high-lift client, of course, wants to be cool or neutral. When a warm result is desired, neutral to slightly cool formulas tone out only part of the natural warmth created.

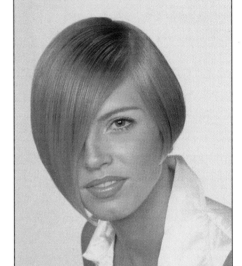

Golden formulas are appropriate in some instances (artificial gold pigment is a cooler, softer gold than the raw-looking gold of lightened natural hair, and some manufacturers' gold series actually have a pretty cool base pigmentation). High-lift beiges are usually slightly warm without being golden (pink-violet).

Color can only lift so much. If you use an 11 level formula on 5 level natural base, you will not get six levels of lift. And the 11 level dyes will be too light to tone out the remaining natural warmth. The result would be raw and untoned. Better you should lift four levels with a formula just four levels lighter—lifting with a 9 level formula would result in a more satisfactory, more thoroughly toned blond on a 5 level natural base. This is **"level-on-level" toning;** the level of the artificial pigment corresponds to the level of underlying natural warmth.

Whatever the stated lifting capability of the product, don't try to exceed it—and if the instructions say to use the target level, do so.

---

1 There is one permanent haircoloring product that uses an "averaging" method of formula selection, but it is the only one of its kind. With this product, you determine the level of color to use by doubling the desired level, and subtracting from this figure the natural level. Say you have a 5 level client that wants to be an 8 level. This is how you select the level to use: 8 + 8 = 16, 16 - 5 = 11. You would use an 11 level formula to achieve an 8 level result, on that 5 level natural base.

No other product is formulated in quite this way, but there are other professional products that use level variance, rather than developer variance, to regulate lift.

Any product which only uses 20 volume developer relies solely on the ammonia content of the tint to vary lightening. Such products do not conform to the principle of lifting with the target level.

The higher the volume of developer, the greater the lift.

Unless instructed otherwise, use the level you wish to achieve (use a 9 level formula to create a 9 level result, for instance).

Natural Base Level

If your client's natural base level falls between levels, err on the safe side and base her formula on the darker of the two. To go the other way is to risk undue warmth. For instance, if a client's natural level is darker than a 4 but lighter than a 3, formulate as though she were a 3.

Very dark natural levels may not lighten a full four or five levels. A client with a natural base of 2 or 3, for instance, may only lift three levels with 40 volume developer.

Texture and Porosity (Condition)

Natural base level primarily determines how light a client can be made in a single process, but texture and tenacity play a part, also. Very coarse, resistant hair is harder to lift than average hair. A client with unusually coarse hair may lift a half-level or a level less than a client with average texture. Very fine hair lifts more readily and is easier to blond. Hair that has been made more porous by previous chemical services will also lighten more readily.

Application and Timing for High-Lift Blonds

Proper virgin application is very important with high-lift blonds (double-application starting ½″ away from the scalp). If first-time high-lift color is applied scalp-to-ends, the result will be uneven. The higher the lift, the greater the disparity—lighter at the scalp area, deeper and more yellow on the cold shaft.

Have a method when you apply color. Some colorists begin by first quartering the hair and applying color on either side of the part lines. Others work in a circular pattern from the crown down. The method you *use* is not as important as *having* a method so your applications will be more consistent and accurate. Taking a lot of thin sections is actually less time-consuming, too, than taking thicker, harder-to-saturate sections (and having to check, recheck, and reapply because the color didn't go on evenly to start with). No matter what the formula, this is good practice, but application errors are more evident with high-lift tint and good technique is extra-important.

High-lift tint should be applied almost as though it were scalp bleach, because it almost is. For a bleach application, the sections are thin enough to see through. On retouches, it is very important to avoid overlapping; exceeding the line of demarcation will result in bands because the overlapped area becomes lighter and more porous. The same is true of high-lift tint.

If there is an area of the hair that is darker, it should be the first to get color. It is not uncommon for a client to be a full level darker in the nape or crown. Begin application of a high-lift formula where the natural level is darkest.

Sometimes a client with otherwise average texture has an extremely fine hairline. The fine hairline will lighten more quickly and, with a very drab formula, it will grab ash. Because it requires less timing, the fine hairline should be the last area of the hair to which the coloring is applied.

Maximum timing ensures maximum toning. To get the most delicate possible tones from your high-lift colors, use the manufacturer's maximum recommended timing the first time you color the hair and on the new growth when you retouch it.

Here is a guideline for ashing out warmth when blonding that works with most color systems:

- When lifting one level, use the neutral (natural) series to contrast-out the warm undertones that will be created (and the appropriate developer, usually 10 or 15 volume).

- When lifting two levels, use an ash series color to neutralize warmth (and the prescribed developer, usually 20 volume).

- When lifting three levels, use an ash series color and a moderate amount of the appropriate ash drabber (usually 30 volume).

- When lifting four levels, use an ash series color and maximum drabber (usually 40 volume).

For maximum lift and toning, most color lines also provide a special high-lift series or blonding boosters.

Colorist's Clipboard

High-lift blonds:

- *Lightening exposes warm natural undertones; contrast-out unwanted warmth with ash.*

- *The majority of color systems instruct you to use the target level when lifting in order to achieve level-on-level toning. Developer volume is varied to regulate lift. (Follow manufacturer's directions.)*

- *Fine hair lifts more readily; coarse hair takes longer and has greater underlying warmth.*

- *Damaged hair lifts more readily and accepts more ash.*

- *Longer timing gives you better toning of underlying warmth.*

- *Utilize proper virgin application.*

- *High-lift colors usually aren't pulled through on retouches. Emulsify the color through ("soapcap") at the shampoo bowl, or use a low- or no-peroxide color to refresh the length.*

- *Don't try to exceed the recommended maximum levels of lift.*

On retouches, repeatedly pulling a high-lift formula through the ends creates unnecessary overporosity and, oftentimes, drab ends. The formula may be pulled through briefly, or emulsified through at the shampoo bowl (wet the hair and massage the color through for a minute or two). It may be necessary to adjust the formula (adding warmth) before it is applied to the length. Rather than pulling the color through, you might refresh the length with a corresponding semi- or demi-permanent, or a color gloss or colored shampoo.

Whenever you are using a drab formula, be especially wary of overporosity. On a virgin application, any overporous ends should be left out initially. The first batch of color would be applied ½″ away from the scalp, through the midshaft, up to where the ends become overporous. Strand testing determines the timing required on overporous ends.

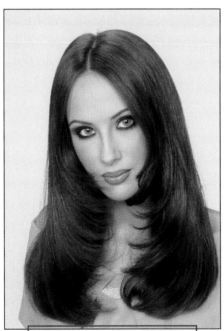

Courtesy of Koger-LaPrairie for Salon JKL.

UNDERSTANDING REDS

Reds have a reputation for being tricky and sensitive, and it's probably well deserved. But once you understand how reds are different, making and maintaining great reds isn't so difficult.

Reds and Porosity

Awareness of porosity is essential in achieving even, true-to-tone reds.

The same red formula on overporous hair will not appear as bright as it would on hair of normal porosity. It is harder to make, and keep, overporous hair red. If a client has overporous ends, you cannot use the same red formula for her ends that you would use for her regrowth—the scalp area would be a nice red, but the ends would be comparatively brown. The formula for overporosity has to be more intense (redder) because overporous hair will tend to show less red. Wherever the hair is overporous, you make the formula redder to start with, adding a brighter red color or intensifying the formula, because overporous hair accepts red tint less readily.

Reds on Gray Hair or Prelightened Hair

Red tint on overporous hair looks drabber (browner), but red tint on gray hair or prelightened hair looks brighter! Red formulas for gray clients are very often muted with a gold or neutral (natural) series. If you ever convert a prelightened client to red tint, be sure to fill properly first in order to get a believable-looking result.

Developer Selection for Reds

Lower volumes used with reds make the tint look deeper and richer (because more natural pigment remains); higher volumes make it look clearer and brighter (because less natural pigment remains and the tint stands alone).

For clients with longer hair, developer strength may be adjusted during a red virgin application to ensure that the length is colored as brightly as the scalp area by using a higher than normal volume (30 rather than 20, for instance) with the initial application on the length (not at the scalp area). This higher volume clears out more natural pigment and achieves a brighter tone on the difficult-to-brighten, hard-keratin length of the hair. This is only done the first time the hair is colored.

When retouching reds, low volumes are used on the length to maintain the condition and brilliance of the hair. Either remix with a low volume, use a low-volume demi-permanent, or dilute the leftover color with water (equal parts) to decrease the volume. Subjecting the length to stronger-than-necessary peroxide damages it unnecessarily, and *damaged hair fades*.

Application and Timing for Reds

As with high-lift blonds, proper virgin application is very important with the reds of permanent haircoloring (double application starting ½″ away from the scalp). The brighter the formula, the more important this is. Scalp-to-ends application will result in a brighter scalp area, guaranteed. (Semi-permanent color is different, and can be applied scalp-to-ends.)

Maximum timing assures maximum deposit, so for the most durable reds, use the product's maximum recommended timing. Reds tend to fade; during retouches the length always needs ample timing, sometimes with a modified formula (a lower volume developer, and/or greater intensity).

Red color clients may be the ones that most benefit from the retouch technique of using per-manent haircoloring on the new growth and a corresponding demi- or semi-permanent on the length. This frequently results in more even color than using oxidative color on the ends, and is usually gentler. Whatever you can do to maintain the *condition* of the hair will also help maintain red pigment in the hair.

Reds and Prepigmenting

Overporous length very often requires filling, to ensure evenness and to prevent fadage. Redheads are more often filled than any other category of color client. When reds fade inordinately, it is a sure sign the hair needs a color filler.

Red tint needs underlying warmth to make it even and durable. (That is what filling supplies.) A natural brunette or brownette will hold red tint better than a natural blond. The hardest hair to keep red is fine, naturally blond hair, or very overporous hair. These are the redheads that will most tend to fade.

Pigmented shampoos or conditioners may be helpful with some red clients, but these are not a substitute for good formulation. Clients who overuse these products will quickly lose the sparkle and believability of their tint.

Reds and Decolorizing

Color removal is probably used more with reds, for a variety of reasons, than with any other type of tinting.

1. **A red client may decide to go brighter, necessitating removal of the brownish cast of the more muted, previously used red tint.**
2. **After repeated retouches with red tint, overporous ends can develop a muddy-looking build-up that needs to be lifted out.**

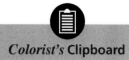

3. **If a red client has a habit of coloring herself between salon visits, her hair will be a rainbow of reds that can only be evened-out by first removing tint.**

4. **A bright red client who wishes to go brown-red (or in any other way significantly change her tone) must first have color removal. The most intense, fashion reds cannot be covered-over; they have to be removed.**

DOUBLE-PROCESS—A PRIMER ON THE USE OF SCALP BLEACH

The lifting capability of single-process haircoloring is limited. Every manufacturer clearly states how many levels of lift is possible with their permanent haircoloring (typically four levels, five in exceptional cases). Beyond that, double-process is necessary: bleach to the desired stage of lightening, then tone, if desired.

First: Assess the Hair and Decide What You Want to Achieve

The key factors that affect the bleach result are the same as for any other haircoloring process: natural level, gray, texture, porosity, and the presence of artificial pigment. More heavily pigmented hair takes longer to lighten; coarse hair takes longer than fine hair; and artificial pigment is harder to lift than natural pigment.

Before you mix your bleach, you must decide exactly what result you want. Consult with your client, as you would for any other color service, to determine the desired level and tone. Then you will know exactly how far to allow the hair to lighten during the bleaching process. If she wants to be a medium

blond, for example, rather than a light blond, you will be leaving more underlying pigment in the hair. Usually, medium blonds need an undertone of gold; light blonds, an undertone of yellow; and very light blonds, pale yellow.

Mixing Scalp Bleach

Mixing bleach to proper consistency has a lot to do with how good your application will be and how efficient the lightening will be. Measure all the ingredients carefully. Pour the developer in first, then the **protinator** (booster), and mix very well—until the crystals dissolve—then put the oil in and mix it well again. The oil thickens it, the developer thins it. You want the bleach to apply in a nice, silky bead—not runny and not pasty. It should stay put, but be wet to the touch so that it lays into the hair properly and doesn't dry out.

Application for Scalp Bleach

The usual method of application for a virgin **bleach-out** is similar to the double-application method for single-process color: first, apply ½″ away from the scalp; then, when the mid-shaft is nearly the desired stage of lightening, apply to the scalp area.

Here is an alternative method of virgin application, shared by Judith Stephens, owner of Sign of the Times in Louisville, Kentucky. First, apply the bleach scalp-to-ends. When the scalp area is the desired stage of lightening, rinse and shampoo. Dry the hair under a cool dryer. Now you can see exactly where the hair needs the second dose of bleach, and you won't have any overlapping or overbleaching of more vulnerable areas of the hair, such as over-porous ends or a fine hairline.

There is no more meticulous application than that for scalp bleach. The rewards for pre-

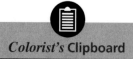

Colorist's Clipboard

Double-process (scalp bleach):

- *The same Universal Method of Formulation that you use for single-process haircoloring applies to double-process.*

- *First, analyze the hair and consult with the client to determine the desired result.*

- *Measure and mix well.*

- *Use proper application technique.*

- *Lift to the natural undertone appropriate for the desired result.*

- *Rinse the bleach and shampoo gently but thoroughly; use an acid rinse before toning.*

cision are even bleaching, even toning, and hair that doesn't break. Begin the application in the darkest or coarsest area of the hair. Take fine sections, thin enough to see through. With retouches, you want no overlapping, of course, and it's easier to avoid overlapping if you just lay a line of bleach at the scalp, then lay the next section against it, rather than smearing the bleach in with your thumb.

If you are lifting past yellow, be patient. Gold is always the toughest pigment color to eliminate. It will probably take longer to go from yellow to pale yellow than it took to bring the natural base to yellow.

Rinsing the Bleach and Preparing the Hair for Toning

With double-process, what you do between the processes is extremely important. When you rinse the bleach, be gentle and thorough. Lukewarm water most efficiently rinses bleach. Do a gentle, thorough shampoo. You might then use an acid rinse or apply some other treatment designed to completely stop the bleaching action. Rinse well and towel dry the hair gently. You may want to use a leave-in porosity treatment. You can then apply your toner on damp hair or dry, as you prefer.

Toners are often oxidative tint. Many companies' permanent haircoloring doubles as a toner, properly selected and used, but a product specifically made for toning will have less ammonia, a lower pH, and in general will be gentler to both the scalp and hair. Toners only need a very low volume developer—the dyes do need to be activated, but that's basically all, as the bleach did the lightening. The purpose of the toner is to conceal or beautify remaining underlying warmth, depositing the desired hue and evening-out small defects in the bleach-out.

The lightest, most delicate toners call for a pale yellow stage of lightening. Lighten too little, leaving yellow still dominant in the hair, and the tone achieved will remain too yellowish. On the other hand, if the toner calls for a yellow stage of lightening, and you overlighten to pale yellow, there will not be enough underlying warmth in the hair to offset the artificial pigment and the hair will display too much of the toner's base color.

How the toner takes depends on porosity, too. Part of the job of the bleach-out is to create the necessary porosity in the hair. Uneven porosity will result in uneven acceptance of the toner, unless the application, timing, or formula is adjusted.

Bobby Jame Hunt

owner of Bobby J's, Pittsburgh, Pennsylvania, talks about an alternative double-process technique:

"If we have someone who is [for example] a 3, and wants to be a 9 level, we'll lift with bleach to a 5 or 6 level—when you see red or orange—then we'll use tint and 40 volume to lift the rest of the way. For the retouch I do the same thing. It works and is less damaging to the hair. We've been doing that for years."

partfour

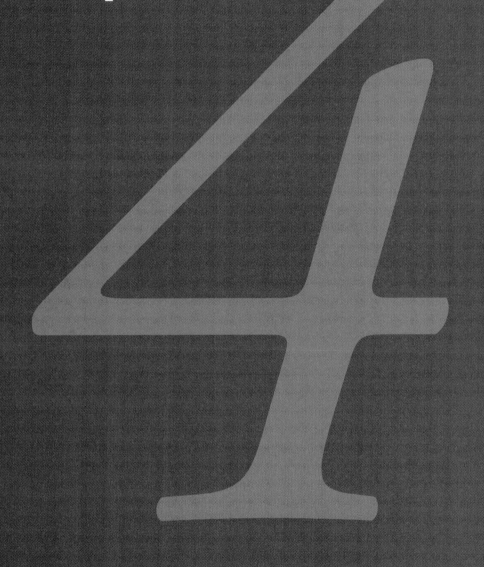

corrective haircoloring

Corrective haircoloring is many things to stylists: a challenge, a great opportunity to win a loyal client, a chance to really help someone and, every so often, it can be just a little scary.

The first chapter in this unit, Chapter Ten, Causes for Corrective Haircoloring, discusses common haircoloring errors as well as unavoidable situations that simply necessitate corrective procedures. This unit begins with an examination of the causes necessitating corrective haircoloring, because prevention, if it is possible, is always preferable to correction. Some corrective work can be avoided; some cannot.

Next, Chapter Eleven, The Universal Method of Formulation Applied to Corrective Haircoloring, puts the emphasis where it has to be in good corrective work (where it has to be in all good haircoloring): on analysis and communication. You cannot correct something until you know what the problem is. The Universal Method of Formulation provides an orderly framework for thinking through corrective cases. This chapter recaps and amplifies the Universal Method of Formulation in terms of corrective haircoloring. The Corrective Troubleshooter on page 111 provides a quick reference for corrective cases; take a look at it whenever you aren't sure how to approach a correction.

Finally, Chapter Twelve, The Corrective Procedures, spells out in detail each subject area categorized as corrective coloring (what it is, when to do it, how to do it): Contrasting-Out Unwanted Tones, Coloring Overporous Hair, Prepigmenting (Color Fillers), Decolorizing (Color Removal), Hair Affected by Minerals, and Hair Affected by Medications.

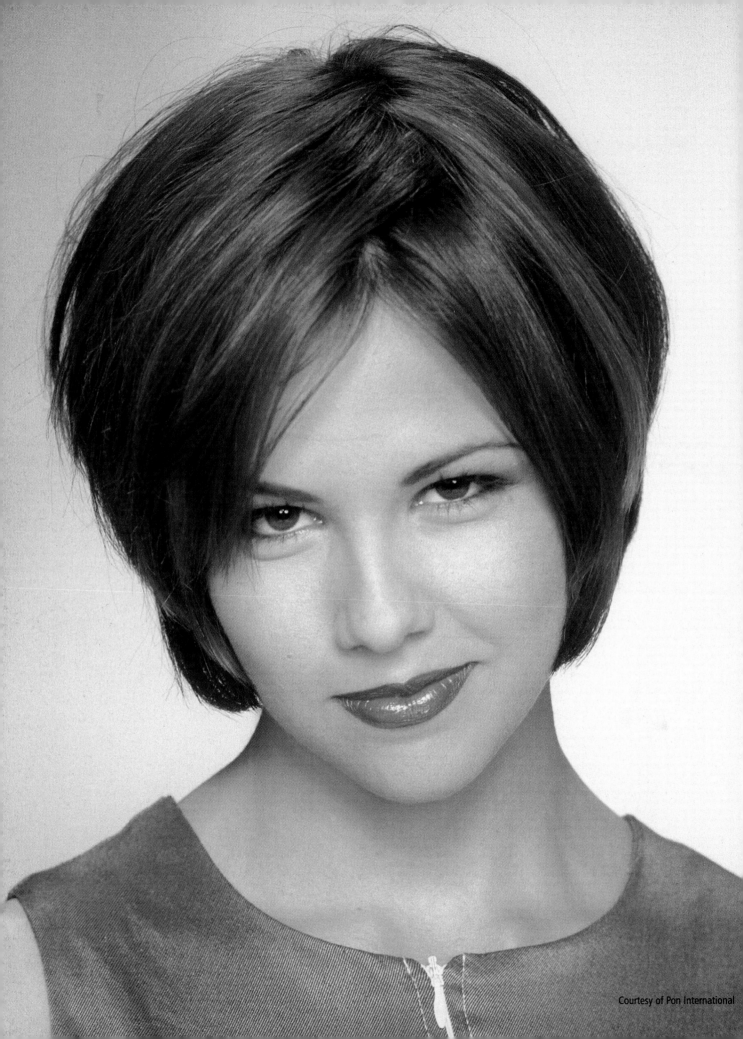

chapter ten

causes for corrective haircoloring

An aware stylist tries not to do things, and discourages her clients from doing things, which ultimately culminate in the need for correction. For every corrective hair-coloring case, there is a set of circumstances that led up to the need for correction, which was sometimes (but not always) avoidable.

Some corrective work can be averted with forethought. In other cases, corrective measures are unavoidable and what matters is your ability to recognize the necessity for prepigmenting, decolorizing, demineralizing, or some other such procedure.

COMMON HAIRCOLORING ERRORS

Miscommunication. Not asking enough questions (or the right questions), or not listening, is the number one cause for corrective coloring. Without all the necessary information, the odds of getting the color right are slim.

Previous tint may be overlooked due to a lack of communication. The condition of the client's hair can be overestimated if a full chemical history isn't taken. Sometimes a client tries to give information about a mineral deposit in her hair, or some other such factor. But, hands-down, the most miscommunicated piece of information is what the client really wants.

What are her expectations? If you don't find out what she wants before you color her hair, you will definitely find out afterwards. You must get the client to show and tell you exactly what she wants.

Insufficient analysis. Neglecting any one of the five key factors spells trouble. Inattention to natural base level, percentage of gray, texture, porosity, or existing tint can all result in an undesirable outcome: too light, too dark, too ash, too brassy, dark or drab ends, an off-cast, and so on. If a color result surprises you, then you missed something in your analysis!

The mishaps that can occur if natural base level isn't taken into account are too numerous to mention—anything can happen if you do not consider the client's natural level—but the most common is unwanted warmth. If percentage of gray is ignored, the result may be too light or off-tone (excessively ash or warm) or the formula may simply fail to cover the gray. Overlook texture, and you may be surprised when coarse hair pulls more warmth or a fine hairline goes dark. If overporosity is overlooked, the color result may be drabber or deeper than expected. If you miss previous tint, the result may be uneven, too dark, or less intense than expected.

Did not read manufacturer's directions. Until you know the color product inside and out, you must rely entirely on the manufacturer's directions. There is no substitute for reading the directions, and no end to the trouble you can get into if you don't read them!

Improper application. The following are the most common application mishaps:

- **Improper retouch of highlighting or frosting clients—repeatedly highlighting the full length of the hair rather than just the regrowth (resulting in overlightened length).**
- **Putting too much color or bleach in foils (resulting in bleeding and bright spots or streaks— "holiday"—at the scalp area).**
- **Improper virgin application with high-lift or reds—scalp-to-ends, instead of a proper double-application (resulting in a lighter or brighter scalp area).**
- **Too thin an application—not enough color used (resulting in poor or spotty lift and deposit, and fadage).**

Improper timing. These are the most common timing mishaps:

- **Did not allow tint to process long enough (gray not covered, high-lift not well-toned, or color fades).**
- **Bleach highlights overprocessed (too light, or white and damaged) or underprocessed (too gold).**

Mistakes Are Part of Learning

There really are no "land mines" in hair, no undetectable elements that will sabotage your efforts! If a color result surprises you, then you missed something in your analysis. If the client's reaction surprises you, then you missed something in the consultation! And if you are sloppy in your application, it may very well tell on you.

All haircolorists have made mistakes; it is part of the learning process. No colorist ever becomes 100 percent infallible, but many do come close. The ones who are close to infallible are the ones who have figured out and learned from their mistakes—accepted them and gone forward.

If you make a mistake, the best thing to do is to acknowledge it. Unless the error is so minute that only you, with your critical eye and desire for perfection, are even aware of the difference, acknowledge the error and take responsibility for it, at least in your own mind.

If you habitually blame someone or something else ("She took an aspirin" / "It's her period" / "Must be on hormones" / "The color machine is acting up" / "It's just the lighting in here" / blah, blah, blah) you will never realize your potential. You do not have to explain the error to your client, but acknowledge it and be honest with yourself. Unless you want to make the same mistake over and over again, you must figure out what happened.

If you fix it, the client will most likely respect and forgive you. She will almost always become more loyal, not less. But, if you send her out the door uncorrected, it is not just one client that has been lost—you have lost potential clients, because negative advertising is more powerful than positive advertising and, moreover, you have lost a piece of your potential. You have lost an opportunity to become more of a colorist and more of a professional. A mistake is a chance to learn.

> **"Dumby: Experience is the name everyone gives to their mistakes.**
>
> **Cecil Graham: One shouldn't commit any.**
>
> **Dumby: Life would be very dull without them."**
>
> —*Oscar Wilde, from* Lady Windermere's Fan.

Colorist's Clipboard

Common haircoloring errors:

- *Lack of communication. You didn't know what she really wanted; she didn't really understand what you were going to do.*

- *Lack of analysis. You forgot to consider porosity, how much gray she has, texture, etc.*

- *You didn't read the manufacturer's directions!*

- *Improper application.*

- *Improper timing.*

Remember, if you make a mistake, everybody makes mistakes—just fix it and learn from it. Try not to make that same mistake again.

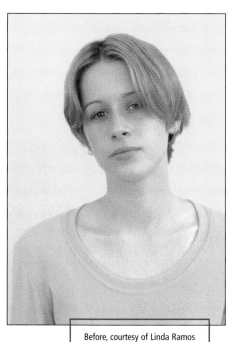

Before, courtesy of Linda Ramos

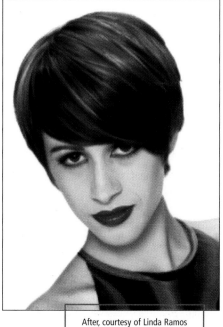

After, courtesy of Linda Ramos

CHANGES IN DESIRED RESULT THAT INVOLVE CORRECTIVE PROCEDURES

Most corrective haircoloring is unavoidable. Corrections may arise because a color client wants a change, or you want to give her a change—to a lighter color, a much darker color, or to a color of a very different tone. What is important in these cases is your ability to recognize the need for corrective procedures. If you have a corrective client in your chair and don't know it, you will expend time, product, and effort doing things that won't work.

A color client wishes to be colored lighter than her existing artificial color. In most cases, you can't just put a lighter tint on her hair. Tint, generally speaking, doesn't lift tint. You will first have to remove the existing artificial color.

A color client wishes to be two or more levels darker than her existing tint. Just applying a darker tint will usually not be enough. To get an even and durable result, you must usually prepigment with some kind of color filler. Going two or three levels darker represents too much of a difference in underlying pigmentation; some of the undertone that was lifted out has to be put back into the hair. Sometimes color filling is advisable even with a single level of deepening, even if it just using a good pigmented shampoo first.

A color client wishes to stay the same level, but wants a significantly different tone. For example, a red-brown color client wishes to be a bright red of the same level, or a bright red color client wishes to go neutral. Although the new formula will be the same level as the existing tint, the tone of the existing color is too different to just be covered up.

Without removing some of the old tint, the result won't be even and tonally correct.

If the client is going darker than the existing tint, you can cover most things up, but drab tint on hair you are trying to make warm may interfere and muddy the result. Very intense reds can be difficult or impossible to cover up and really must be decolorized.

A double-process or heavily highlighted client wishes to convert to high-lift tint. The previously bleached hair must be filled. High-lift tint will not lighten the hair as much as bleach did; the previously bleached hair will have to be deepened, and filled first to get the tint to take evenly and hold. The formula for the regrowth will be completely different from the formula for the lightened length. The length is overporous and lacks underlying pigment, whereas the regrowth must be lifted and its underlying warmth reduced.

OTHER CAUSES

Simple neglect. Damaged hair fades. A client who damages her hair, or allows it to become damaged, will battle fadage and require special formulation. Certain shampoos and conditioners may strip color, as well. And waiting too long between touch-ups may make the next color appointment more involved.

She colored her own hair. The client who cannot resist coloring her own hair frequently requires correction. Home haircoloring looks so easy on the TV commercials; some clients find out firsthand it's not so easy.

Mineral build-up in the hair. In some places this is a constant problem. The water supply in such areas has a heavy mineral load that results in build-ups and possible chemical failures. In other regions, the water is

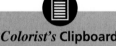

Colorist's Clipboard

Changing a client's existing artificial haircoloring may require corrective procedures:

- Going lighter than the existing artificial color,

- Going more than two levels deeper, or

- Changing the tone of the haircoloring very much.

relatively mineral free and build-ups are rarely seen, but regardless of location, we all deal occasionally with **swimmer's hair** ("chlorine green").

Metallic tint on the hair. Metallic salts are incompatible with oxidation chemicals. Neither oxidizing tint nor bleach can be used safely on hair treated with metallic tint, and a special neutralizer must be used in perming (**sodium bromate** rather than hydrogen peroxide). Few salon clients ever use such products (because their stylist tells them not to!).

Hair affected by medications. In rare instances, hair texture or condition may be affected by illness or by certain drugs, and this then influences how the colorist proceeds. The most common problem related to illness or medicine is increased dryness and porosity.

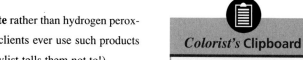

Colorist's Clipboard

Other factors that make correction necessary:

• *The client's hair becomes damaged, or she waits too long between retouches.*

• *She colored her hair herself.*

• *Mineral build-up from using swimming pools or a high mineral content in her water at home.*

• *Illness or medicine has affected the condition of her hair.*

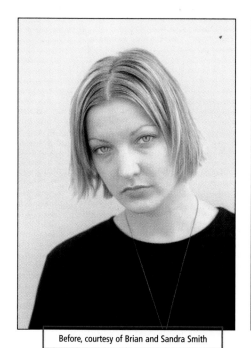

Before, courtesy of Brian and Sandra Smith

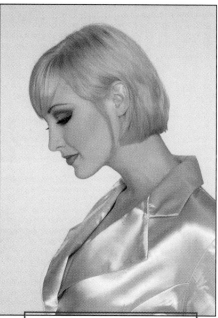

After, courtesy of Brian and Sandra Smith

Courtesy of Hugo / Heather Solana for Sculpt Salon

the universal method of formulation applied to corrective haircoloring

Corrective haircoloring, like all haircoloring, is based entirely on basic color principles. A stylist learning corrective haircoloring will experience a renewed appreciation for the basics. It is the most experienced colorists who have the deepest regard for the basic laws of color.

The Universal Method of Formulation, which is derived from the basic laws of haircoloring, applies to all haircoloring, including corrective work.

Norman Zapien, a long-time salon owner in Atlanta, Georgia, puts it like this: "Basic is advanced. What does it take to get basic? It takes a lot of tearing things apart. You have to be advanced to get basic."

Only through careful analysis and communication can the problem(s) be identified and a course of action planned. You cannot fix a color if you do not know what is wrong with it. Analysis and communication clarify what the problem actually is, or what the problems are, making it possible to identify the solution(s).

CONSULTING WITH CORRECTIVE CLIENTS

Have you ever stood over a corrective client and thought to yourself, "Man! Where do I start?!"

What makes corrective heads seem complicated is that there is usually a lot going on, more than one set of key factors. The new growth, midshaft, and ends may all be different. There are multiple porosities and different levels and tones of tint; different areas of the hair *are* different.

So where do you start?

You start by first asking the client about her hair ("Tell me about your hair") to find out from her what it is she doesn't like, even if you think you already know.

Then you analyze each area of her hair: new growth, midshaft, and ends, front to back. This will clarify for you what the problem really is.

Assessing a Corrective Case

Look at the hair at the scalp area. Identify the key factors there (it may be new growth or freshly colored): natural level, percentage of gray, texture, porosity, and existing tint. If the hair is freshly colored and this is the client's first visit to your salon, you will have to make an intelligent estimate of her natural base level.

Then examine the length of the hair. Identify the key factors for the midshaft, and then for the ends. Be especially alert to over-porosity. Use your swatches to identify the level(s) of the previous tint, and note its tone(s). Find out what type of haircoloring was previously used.

Analysis brings order to chaos. It brings the real problem(s) into focus and makes the case manageable. Reread Chapter Four: Analyzing the Hair (pages 45–50). The method of analysis is exactly the same for the corrective client (it is the same for all clients, all types of haircoloring, all products).

Communicating with the Corrective Client

Even if it seems obvious, ask the client to state for you what she finds objectionable about her haircoloring. Then determine exactly what color result she wants, in terms of level and tone. Reread Chapter Five, Communicating with the Client (pages 53–60). Clients do not describe colors the way colorists do. A thousand words are not enough to be sure that your client is thinking what you are thinking. She must *show* you what she wants, using swatches or other visuals.

Once you have determined what she wants, and what is appropriate for her, estimate for her the cost of today's services. Tell her when you are likely to need to see her again and what future appointments will probably involve; corrective cases often require more maintenance. Let her know that you are *striving* for perfection, that today's result will be *good* and that it will become *more perfect* with each coloring.

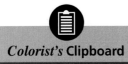

Colorist's Clipboard

Consulting with corrective clients:

- Take time to do a thorough analysis of the client's hair; write down what you see.

- Be extra careful in your communication; be sure you and the client understand each other.

- Use the Universal Method of Formulation to clarify what the problem is.

I. In general, what is it about her color she wants corrected?

_____

_____

_____

II. Assess the Key Factors

Natural level = _____

Percentage of gray = _____

Texture = _____

Porosity:

New growth = _____

Midshaft = _____

Ends = _____

Existing tint:

What level is it?

New growth = _____

Midshaft = _____

Ends = _____

What tone is it?

New growth = _____

Midshaft = _____

Ends = _____

What type(s) of haircoloring is on her hair? _____

_____

III. Exactly what color do you want to achieve—target level(s) and tone(s)?

_____

_____

IV. What do you have to do to achieve the desired result at the:

New growth?_____

_____

_____

Midshaft?_____

_____

_____

Ends? _____

_____

_____

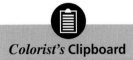

Consultation format for corrective coloring:

- Corrective cases call for an emphasis on client communication and proper analysis.

- Thoroughly analyze the client's hair, noting the key factors for new growth, midshaft, and ends.

- Pay close attention to porosity and previous tint.

- Determine what the client really wants, by actively listening.

- What is it she doesn't like about her current color?

- What is the desired end result?

- What procedures will produce that desired result?

Checklist: The Universal Method of Formulation Applied to Corrective Coloring

1. Analysis (analyze new growth, midshaft, and ends):
- ❑ What is the client's natural base level?
- ❑ Percentage of gray?
- ❑ Texture?
- ❑ Porosity?
- ❑ What level is the existing tint?

2. Communication
- ❑ What end result does the client have in mind?
- ❑ What tint has been previously used, and when?
- ❑ What range of levels and tones best suit her?
- ❑ How much maintenance is she capable of?
- ❑ What procedures do you recommend?

Pinpoint the desired end result by level and tone.

3. Formulation

A haircoloring result is the combined effect of the key factors and the formula used.

Key Factors + Formula = Result
- ❑ Given her key factors, what procedures and formulas will produce the desired result for the:
  - a. new growth?
  - b. midshaft?
  - c. ends?
- ❑ Select the appropriate procedures and formulas per manufacturer's directions. Measure and mix per directions, strand testing as necessary.

4. Application
- ❑ Any necessary corrective procedures are done first.
- ❑ Timing is determined by strand testing.

The problem will be one, or a combination of, the following:

1. **Wrong level: too light or too dark**
2. **Wrong tone: too warm (too much red, orange, or gold) or too drab (not enough warmth; an off-cast)**
3. **Uneven color: drab ends, dark ends, dark hairline, holiday (bright spots or gaps), demarcation or bands, or bright scalp area.**
4. **Gray did not cover**
5. **Fadage**

The solution will be one, or a combination of, the following:

1. **Wrong level:**

If she is *too light*, you will be making her darker (possibly prepigmenting first).

If she is *too dark*, you will be making her lighter. (Oxidizing tints are lightened by decolorizing or bleaching, other types of dyes may require a different procedure. You must find out what type of haircoloring is on her hair, and the brand name, if possible.)

2. **Wrong tone:**

Too warm: contrast-out the unwanted warmth, for reds, possible decolorizing.

Too ash: contrast-out the unwanted ash (possible decolorizing).

Off-casts: consider the source of the cast—if it's caused by haircoloring, remove or contrast-out.

For *overporosity*, add warmth to the formula.

Off-casts caused by minerals (the orange of iron or swimmer's green): use a good demineralizing treatment; if necessary, contrast-out any remaining cast.

3. **Uneven color:**

Drab ends: contrast-out or remove color.

Dark ends or hairline: remove color.

Bright spots (foils bled): use the natural level to cover-up any bright spots.

Gaps in the application: apply the same formula to any spots that were missed.

Demarcations or bands: blend the imperfections, deepening if too light, lightening if too deep.

Bright scalp area: contrast-out the undue brightness.

4. **Gray not covered:**

Adjust the formula, application, and timing to maximize coverage (possible presoftening or prepigmentation).

5. **Fadage:**

Increase timing and/or prepigment, consider after-care.

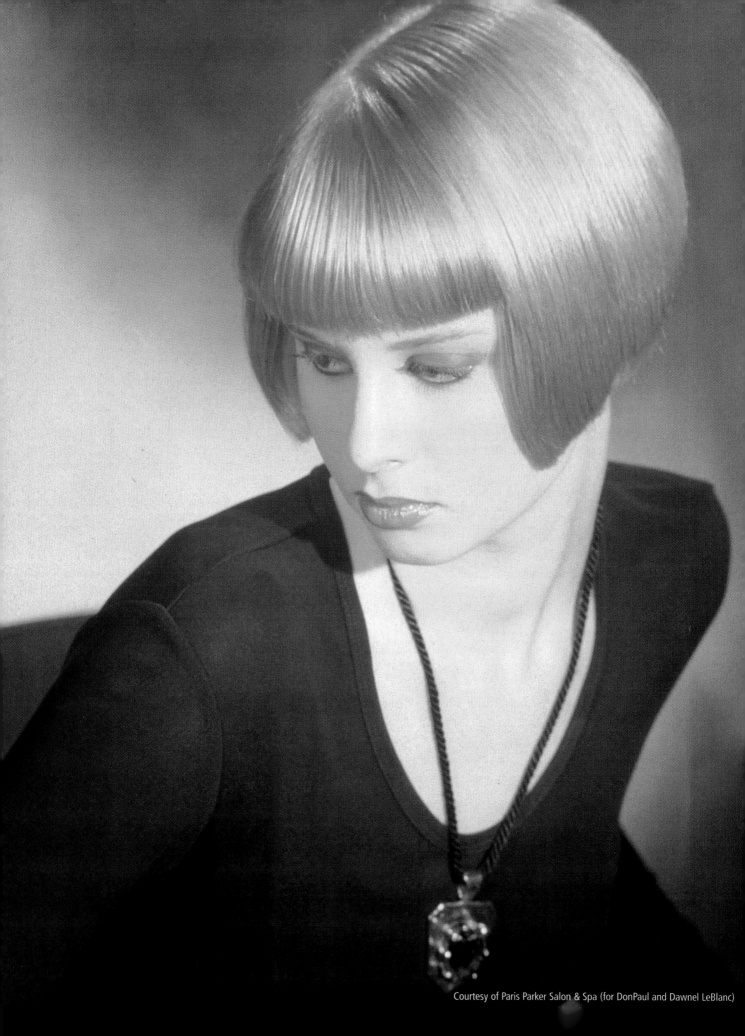

Courtesy of Paris Parker Salon & Spa (for DonPaul and Dawnel LeBlanc)

the corrective procedures

Corrective haircoloring consists of these subject areas: Contrasting-Out Unwanted Tones, Coloring Overporous Hair, Prepigmenting (Color Fillers), Decolorizing (Color Removal), Hair Affected by Minerals, and Hair Affected by Medications.

Corrective haircoloring is mastered through experience. Once you begin doing it, it makes more sense and ceases to be intimidating. Do enough of it and you learn the fine points that really cannot be conveyed in any other way; you develop a feel for it, in other words.

Knowledge of basic coloring is what guides the colorist through any corrective case. You have already read everything that corrective haircoloring is based upon, in the preceeding chapters. Corrective haircoloring is simply an extension of basic haircoloring.

Michael Burton

haircolorist and owner
of Michael Burton Colors
in Atlanta, Georgia:

"You are only as good as your

ability to repair your worst

mistake, on the spot."

Contrasting formulas, used

to mute unwanted tones,

are based on the principle

of complementary pairs.

CONTRASTING-OUT UNWANTED TONES

Unwanted tones are neutralized by using the color wheel concept of contrasting colors, or complementary pairs. In some cases, the unwanted color should be lifted out of the hair instead of contrasted-out.

Unwanted tones consist of either too much warmth or too much ash.

Common instances of excessive warmth include: a high-lift client whose formula did not have enough ash in it, a client with a dark natural base that you try to lift more than tint can take her, a high-lift client whose color fades to brass, sunlightened clients, and clients lightened by perming. Any time natural pigment is lightened, accidentally or by design, warmth is created. These cases are corrected by ashing-out the unwanted warmth, using a cool formula of the client's existing level. For example, if your client's sunlightened ends are an 8 level gold, you would use an 8 level cool formula to contrast-out the unwanted warmth.

When hair is too ash, warmth neutralizes it (although sometimes it is better to lift the ash cast out, partly or completely). Ash haircoloring can go drab on overporous ends; on gray hair it can go drab or off-tone. In such cases you might color right over the ash cast with a warm formula. If the ash cast is also a little dark, though, you would first need to lift some of the deposit with a mild decolorizer.

Ash contrasts-out warmth, and vice-versa. Contrasting formulas, used to mute unwanted tones, are based on the principle of complementary pairs: opposites on the color wheel neutralize each other. If a client's hair is too warm, a natural or ash formula will neutralize it, or "brown-it-out" (make it a neutral tone, which is

brown or beige). If the unwanted warmth is gold, then violet will best neutralize it. Orange, which is commonly called "brassiness," is best browned-out with a blue-based color.

The level of the contrasting formula should generally correspond to the level of the cast you are trying to eliminate. This is called **level-on-level toning.** If you try to contrast-out an unwanted tone using a paler formula, it will have minimal or no effect. The two have to be the same lightness or depth. (A 9 level ash formula used to tone a 7 level brassy head will have little effect, but a 7 level formula will mute the brass.)

If an unwanted cast is too dark, the solution is not toning, but color removal. Whenever tint is too dark, it needs to be lifted-out, not covered up. Because excessive ashiness is usually caused by artificial tint, it may be better to lift the tint rather than trying to contrast it out. Especially with lighter levels, drab artificial pigment under warm pigment can look muddy; lifting the drab cast first gives a more natural-looking result. Contrasting colors "brown-out" each other. If you are trying to create a bright red or a delicate, irridescent blond, you don't want brown, so lifting-out is a better option than contrasting-out. Then you have a clean slate upon which to deposit the desired tone.

Minerals can also be a source of unwanted casts. A client with "swimming-pool green" or an iron-orange cast should be demineralized, to eliminate the discoloration and the mineral as much as possible, before using a contrasting color.

COLORING OVERPOROUS HAIR

Uneven porosity can cause an uneven result, because overporous hair accepts artificial pigment differently. There are different ways to compensate for overporosity—the formula, how you apply, or the processing time can all be adjusted. The formula may be intensified, or made warmer, and a lower volume developer used. The hair may be dampened with water before coloring, or with a leave-in treatment, to help equalize it. You might use a color filler of some kind. Timing may be very brief, because overporous hair processes fast.

Adjusting the Formula

Overporous hair accepts oxidation dyes selectively; when you are using permanent haircoloring, especially, overporous hair tends to reject warmth and accept ash. The more overporous it is, the more it selects-out warmth and grabs ash, which is termed "abused rejection."

For example: red tint pulled through overporous ends without adjustment will not be as bright. The ends will appear more muted and neutral (browner or with blond levels, tan or washed-out), and overporous ends may go darker, too. What do you do? You intensify the retouch formula before applying it to the ends—add some brighter red to the existing tint (maybe a little, maybe a lot, depending on the degree of overporosity). The overporous hair will reject red, and absorb whatever brown it can find in the formula, so you allow for that by making the formula for the ends redder to start with. Strand test to determine how much brighter the formula has to be.

For overporous ends, you can either add extra warmth (red or gold) to the existing formula before pulling it through, or mix an entirely different, warmer formula, using a low volume developer. A semi- or demi-permanent product is often an excellent choice for overporous ends.

An ash formula intended to contrast-out warmth when lifting will easily go drab and deep on overporous ends. When a retouch formula is very drab, a completely different formula should be used on overporous ends. Depending on the tone desired, degree of fadage, and degree of overporosity, this formula may be neutral, slightly warm, or quite warm, and it might also need to be a level lighter. Strand test when formulating for overporosity.

Some color systems have drabber bases than others and require more adjustment. Others require adjustment only in the most extreme cases. Manufacturers print guidelines for coloring overporous hair and intensifying formulas in their literature, or will provide this information over the phone. Once you really know the tones of the haircoloring product you are working with, you will be able to closely judge what overporous hair requires.

Lowering the Volume

Hair which is overporous and already lightened needs only a weak developer, just enough to activate the dyes—10 volume is often ideal. Semi-permanent haircoloring and no-ammonia demi-permanents are good choices to refresh overporous length because they provide deposit without lift.

Other ways to lower the volume when you are pulling color through is to add an equal part of water to the leftover color, or to wet the length at the shampoo bowl and emusify the color through briefly. When you add water to permanent haircoloring you drop the **working volume** of the formula.

When lightening overporous hair, expect it to lift more readily than hair of normal porosity. A weaker formula will do—use a lower volume and don't make it as ashy.

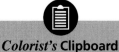

Colorist's Clipboard

Contrasting-out unwanted tones:

- *An unwanted tone is neutralized by its complement (the color opposite it—directly across from it—on the color wheel).*

- *Ash contrasts-out warmth, and warmth contrasts-out ash.*

- *These are the contrasting pairs:*
  1. *Violet and Yellow*
  2. *Orange and Blue*
  3. *Green and Red*
  4. *Yellow-Orange and Blue-Violet*
  5. *Yellow-Green and Red-Violet*
  6. *Red-Orange and Blue-Green*

- *In some cases, color removal may be a better remedy (when the cast is also too dark, or when a brown or tan deposit would interfere with the desired end result).*

- *Hair that is off-tone due to minerals should be demineralized first, then colored with a contrasting formula if necessary.*

Applying to Damp Hair

With overporous hair, it is usually easier to apply color damp, rather than dry. The color goes on more easily and evenly. You can either use a water bottle to dampen the overporous length, or lightly preshampoo beforehand.

Filling (Prepigmenting)

In cases of extreme overporosity or continued fadage, a color filler is necessary. Hair that just doesn't color evenly in a single step or fades excessively needs to be prepigmented.

Timing on Overporous Hair

On overporous hair, timing is determined by strand testing.

If the regrowth is normal but the length is overporous (which is almost always the situation), get the color on the new growth and test the length while it is processing. On overporous hair, timing is normally brief—five minutes or less to refresh, ten or 15 minutes to really deposit.

PREPIGMENTING (COLOR FILLERS)

Maybe you have heard it said, "Anything is a filler—water is a filler; it fills the hair—anything will fill the hair!" It's true that hair will absorb any liquid, becoming "filled," but color fillers do more than just saturate hair.

In a way, we do employ water as a filler with overporous clients. Many colorists spritz overporous hair with water before a color application, to help distribute the color more evenly through the damaged areas. Some colorists add water to tint before pulling it through the ends.

So is water a filler?

Is a conditioner a filler? Some treatments are designed to even out porosity—fill in the overporous areas, lay down the cuticle, and

buffer the damaged spots. This type of conditioner does enhance the feel of the hair, and can even make a difference in the evenness of the color result, but it is not a substitute for a color filler.

Color fillers have a very specific purpose, one which only dyes, and only the right dyes, can fulfill. *The purpose of color fillers is to replace missing underlying warmth and compensate for overporosity.* A color filler replaces missing underlying pigment, providing the substructure for the tint which is then applied over it.

For example: a medium-brown tint client is very overporous and visibly lighter on her length. A light red filler, thinly applied to the overporous ends before coloring, will help ensure an even and durable color result. Without that base of appropriate warmth, the brown haircoloring would tend to take unevenly and fade.

A **color filler** provides the necessary base pigmentation to support and maintain tint, making even color deposit possible and averting fadage on overporous or overlightened hair.

When Is a Color Filler Necessary?

It is appropriate to prepigment hair:

1. **When overporous ends take color unevenly or tend to fade.**
2. **When a tint client wishes to be significantly deeper than her existing color (usually two or more levels darker).**
3. **Whenever permanent haircoloring fades excessively.**

How common is very overporous hair in your salon? Overlightened hair? Fadage? *That's* how common filling should be.

Prepigmenting recommendations vary from manufacturer to manufacturer. Techniques vary a little from colorist to colorist,

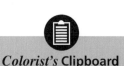

Colorist's Clipboard

Coloring overporous hair:

• *Overporous hair processes faster and tends to go drabber and deeper with permanent haircoloring.*

• *Use a shorter timing.*

• *Use more warmth (less ash).*

• *Use a weak developer.*

• *Consider prepigmenting.*

• *Determine the formula and timing by strand testing.*

• *With semi-permanent haircoloring, overporous areas of the hair will be brighter. If this is undesirable, mute the formula for the overporous area by adding a neutral or gold tone.*

too; you may want to look over your colleagues' shoulders to see what products and methods they like to use.

Selecting Color Fillers

Color fillers are haircoloring. Permanent haircoloring is often used as a filler. Many demi- and semi-permanents can be used as color fillers and are superb as such. In some cases, a few washes with a good colored shampoo is sufficient to fill. Some companies make haircoloring products specifically to be used as fillers and these are excellent. Read manufacturers' directions and try different products and techniques; you will develop different ways of filling for different situations.

The filling recommendations in your manufacturer's literature will almost parallel an underlying pigment chart, because it is the purpose of fillers to replace missing underlying warmth. Color fillers are always warm.

How do you know what color to fill with? *Color fillers are slightly lighter than the underlying pigment of the color you want to achieve,* depending on the tonal result desired, porosity, and the product used.

The filler for a dark blond, for instance, would be light orange to dark gold (light orange for a red blond result, dark gold for a neutral result). For a light brown, the filler would be dark to light orange; for a medium brown, red to dark orange.

General Guidelines for Prepigmenting

1. **Follow manufacturer's directions regarding filler selection, application, timing, and rinsing or blotting.**
2. **A filler should be applied only to the area of the hair that needs it,**
   not all over—only where over-porosity, overlightening, or fadage dictates.
3. **Application of a filler is not as heavy as a color application. A filler is a thin veil, only enough to evenly stain the hair. Fillers are generally more-liquid mixtures, applied lightly but worked into the hair thoroughly.**
4. **When permanent haircoloring is used to fill, a very low-volume developer is used and processing time is usually half or a third that of normal timing. You may be instructed to rinse off the filler, or to blot it, or to apply the tint right over it.**
5. **Color fillers are always warm. Ash tint is generally not advisable over a filler. To get the coolest possible result, a lighter filler is used (gold with just a little orange in it, for instance, instead of orange) with a natural (neutral) series formula applied over it. If the end result is undesirably warm, the filler used was too dark or intense.**

Filling and Tinting-Back

Tinting-back means putting the depth back into chemically lightened hair.

A **tint-back** returns to the hair what lightening took out, starting with the warm underlying pigment, in the form of a color filler. Tinting-back is usually a two-step service: first prepigment, then deepen.

For instance: you wish to tint a previously bleached client light brown; the first step

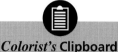

Colorist's **Clipboard**

Prepigmenting:

• *The purpose of a color filler is to replace missing underlying warmth and compensate for overporosity:*

  1. *When overporous ends take color unevenly or fade,*

  2. *When a tint client wants to be two or more levels darker than her existing color, or*

  3. *Whenever color fades excessively.*

• *Color fillers are always warm and usually slightly lighter than the undertone of the desired level.*

would be to fill the bleached hair, using a reddish gold (light orange) formula, slightly lighter than the dominant underlying pigment of light brown. Without that filler, the light brown haircoloring would take unevenly and would quickly fade.

Tinting-back doesn't always mean a return to the client's natural base level. In fact, previously lightened clients usually don't want to be as dark as they are (or were) naturally—it's too extreme a change. Tint-backs more typically involve darkening a bleach or high-lift client two or three levels. If you are deepening only a couple of levels, you can sometimes skip the filler and just use a demi-permanent color, formulating lighter and warmer to adjust for porosity.

If the client's hair already displays strong warmth, filling is probably not necessary. When tinting back, determine how many levels deeper the client wants to be, and then decide whether or not there is already adequate warmth in the hair to maintain that level of depth.

Maintaining Tint-Backs

Tint-backs tend to fade. Proper application and formulation minimize fadage, but a tint-back will still fade sooner than the average tint application. The trick to getting a tint-back to hold is to have the client return for another application (filler and tint) *before* the tint-back has a chance to fade considerably. Have the client schedule another color appointment for no more than three weeks from the date of the initial tint-back. Two weeks may be better if she plans to spend time in the sun or does other things that promote rapid fadage.

If you put more pigment into the hair while the original tint-back is still mostly there, you begin getting a more normal build-up of pigment, which will then really hold. If you allow the tint-back to fade, you are back to square one with the client. Tint-back clients may benefit more than anyone from a good colored shampoo or conditioner.

A client with excessively highlighted hair who wants her **corrective lowlighting** to last cannot treat the lowlighting as though it were a

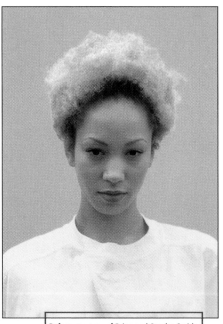

Before, courtesy of Brian and Sandra Smith.

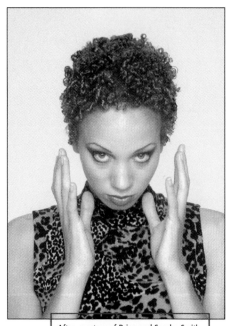

After, courtesy of Brian and Sandra Smith.

highlighting, thinking she won't need maintenance for two or three months. If she really wants a long-term correction, she needs to return to the salon before her lowlighting disappears—within the month. Most lowlighting (reverse-frost) clients are content, though, to allow the shading to gradually disappear, and have some lowlights added when their highlighting is retouched.

DECOLORIZING (COLOR REMOVAL)

Artificial haircoloring is lightened by **color removal,** or **decolorizing.** As a general rule, tint does not lift tint, and tint does not lift any other type of haircoloring, either. Permanent haircoloring lightens natural pigment; it generally does not lighten artificial pigment of any kind.

Color removal was once called "stripping the hair" (a decolorizer was a **stripper**), an unbeautiful term that evokes images of devastated hair. We now say *decolorizing* or *color removal.*

Types of Decolorizers

When we talk about color removers, most of the time we are talking about products intended to remove oxidation tint. Color removers designed to lift oxidation tint are almost always bleaches (mild bleaches, milder than scalp bleach). They are formulated to be gentle and leave the hair in the best possible condition. There is a good selection of color-removing bleaches available, but some colorists prefer to use scalp or highlighting bleaches instead, mixed with low-volume developers or just water. *If a color remover can be mixed with hydrogen peroxide, it must be considered bleach; it is capable of lightening natural pigment as well as dyes, even if you only mix it with water.*

Another type of remover for permanent haircoloring consists of **reducing agents** that unravel the dye molecules in the hair, rather than lightening by bleaching. This type is far less commonly available. Once the desired degree of decolorizing is achieved, the hair is neutralized with a low volume of hydrogen peroxide. (Permanent waving, another reducing process, also uses hydrogen peroxide neutralization.) This type of decolorizer is effective only with oxidation tint, as it does not lighten direct dyes, and it does not lighten natural pigment.

Color removers for semi-permanent products are generally oil-based **solvents.** When it is necessary to remove anything other than permanent haircoloring, it is wise to ask the manufacturer of the product you want to remove about the recommended means of removal.

When Is Decolorizing Necessary?

Color removal is necessary whenever a color client wants to be lighter than her existing tint. Haircoloring is lightened with a decolorizer, not by applying lighter haircoloring.

Color removal may also be necessary when a color client wants a much different tone, even though she is not going lighter. Drab tint on hair you are trying to make warm can interfere and muddy the result, and really should be lifted out. Likewise, intense warmth can be difficult to cover up and really should be removed.

Removal of Temporary and Semi-Permanent Haircoloring

Sometimes these are removed with bleach, but there is an equal chance that the manufacturer will recommend some other method. A "semi-permanent" which is really an oxidizing tint (a

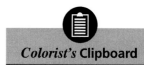

Colorist's **Clipboard**

Decolorizing:

- *When a color client wants to go lighter than her existing tint, or wants a very different tone, color removal is necessary.*

- *As a general rule, tint does not lift tint.*

- *Temporary and semi-permanent products have different dye systems and may require a method of removal different from permanent haircoloring.*

demi-permanent) will probably be removed the same way you remove permanent haircoloring—with bleach—but always check with the manufacturer. Many temporary and semi-permanent products utilize dyes that are very resistant to bleaching, and if you use a bleach-type remover, all you will succeed in doing is lightening the natural pigment, and possibly drive the dyes further into the hair.

The best advice on this subject is: *Consult the manufacturer of the product you wish to remove, and follow their advice.* Methods of removal are as diverse as the temporary and semi-permanent categories—and temporary and semi-permanent products vary widely. Treatment with an oily mixture is a typical recommendation for removal of semi-permanent haircoloring, and for most coating products (saturate the hair with the oil treatment, cover with a plastic cap, and process under a warm dryer). An alkaline shampoo or a clarifying treatment may reduce the intensity of some dyes (these are also usually processed with heat). Sometimes bleaching is recommended. But don't assume that because one temporary or semi-permanent product is removed a certain way that others will be, too. To avoid wasting time, and to possibly avoid needless damage to the hair, check the manufacturer's literature or call their toll-free phone number. After all, nobody knows a product better than the company that created it.

With certain products, only so much removal is possible and covering up the deposit may be a more effective option.

Removal of Metallic Tint

Lead acetate is by far the most common metallic dye. Professional products do not contain metallic salts and salon clients rarely use metallic products. In addition to reactivity with salon chemicals, they are generally dulling and unnatural-looking. Products containing lead acetate are marketed strictly for home use. The consumer repeatedly applies the tint to her hair, daily at first, until enough lead accumulates to color the gray satisfactorily.

Makers of metallic dye products caution against the use of oxidization color, bleach, or hydrogen peroxide neutralizers on hair that has metallic color on it.

To remove a metallic dye, follow the advice of the manufacturer, strand testing first. The recommended method of removal is likely to be a very, very weak hydrogen peroxide shampoo. The truth is that there are not many metallic products left; one very famous company dominates the lead acetate market, and while hennas have been known to be adulterated with metallic salts (and you might exercise caution if your client has used a henna with which you are unfamiliar), the most popular hennas are pure vegetable products that can be safely treated with bleach-type decolorizers.

Does this ring a bell: the **1:20 test** for metals? Mix *one* ounce of clear 20 volume H_2O_2 and *20* drops of household ammonia; snip a hair sample from the client and insert it in the solution. Hair with lead acetate on it lightens much, much faster than would hair colored with oxidation tint.

How to Begin a Decolorizing Service

Conduct a proper analysis and consultation (refer back to Chapters Four and Five). Be sure to establish what type of haircoloring is on the hair, obtaining the brand name if possible, so that you can determine the appropriate means of removal. Determine the level and tone of the color you want to achieve. In cases of an espe-

Don't assume that because one temporary or semi-permanent product is removed a certain way that others will be, too.

cially heavy build-up or a product you are unfamiliar with, it is best to avoid making promises upfront about the level you will achieve today.

Remember:

1. **The target level and tone determine how much removal is necessary.**
2. **The degree of removal necessary, and the quality of the hair, determine how strong a solution to use.**

Determining How Much to Lighten

The target level and tone determine how much lightening is necessary. You will need to decolorize slightly beyond the dominant underlying color of the level you want to achieve. For example, if the desired level is a light brown, you will be decolorizing to the light orange stage. If the desired tone were red, you would leave a little more pigment in the hair, decolorizing to dark orange (see Table 12-1).

General Guidelines for Color Removal

1. A color remover which is bleach will lift natural as well as artificial pigment. Almost all products designed to remove permanent haircoloring are actually mild bleaches, which will also lighten natural pigment. Apply decolorizers only to the part of the hair that needs decolorizing, to avoid unnecessary lightening of virgin areas.

2. For more effective removal which is also kinder to the hair, begin with a weaker rather than a stronger solution—the weakest appropriate solution, given the tint build-up. This allows you to "read" the hair. The tint may lift more quickly than expected, or it may lift very unevenly. Spotty lift is typical; where there is a greater build-up of tint in the hair, due to porosity, repeated application, or overlapping, the tint will be more tenacious. A mild initial application allows you to discover where the tint deposit is more stubborn without drastically overlightening the rest of the hair.

3. Consider how many layers (applications) of tint the client has on her hair. The heavier the build-up of tint, the longer removal will take, and stronger solutions will be required. If there is only an application or two of tint, it will lighten much more readily, and a weaker solution will suffice.

4. Bleach-type decolorizers can be mixed with various volumes of hydrogen peroxide, or just with water, or even diluted with shampoo, to vary the strength and speed of lightening.

Desired Level	Dominant Underlying Color	Decolorize To
Light Blond	Yellow (light gold)	pale yellow
Medium Blond	Gold	yellow
Dark Blond	Reddish Gold (light orange)	gold
Light Brown	Golden Red (dark orange)	light orange
Medium Brown	Red	dark orange
Dark Brown	Red Brown	red

TABLE 12-1   DECOLORIZATION GUIDE

*If the color result is to be beared, decolorize only to the dominent undertone of the desired level, leaving greater underlying warmth in the hair.

5. Lighter levels of tint lift more easily than darker levels. Light brown haircoloring lightens more easily than dark brown, and dark brown lightens more easily than black. Very dark tint may only lighten so much before the hair is compromised unacceptably. Black tint, for instance, may only lighten to a red stage after continued bleaching. With dark tint and some staining products it is best to make no promises but to allow the hair to speak for itself.

6. A color remover is thinner than other forms of bleach, so that it can be rapidly applied. If you mix a scalp or highlighting bleach for decolorizing, mix it wet and thin.

7. Always begin application of any color remover in the back of the head. If the tint lightens faster than anticipated, you can lay the client back in the shampoo bowl and rinse where you applied first, allowing the front to catch up.

8. Stay away from the scalp area initially. It will lighten much more readily than the midshaft and ends. Not only does it have the benefit of body heat, but in most cases the hair closest to the scalp has been exposed to much less tint. The ends normally have the toughest build-up. With long hair, the midshaft is often slowest to lift.

9. Color removal has no set timing. It takes as long as it takes, so watch it carefully. Leave the remover on until the desired lightening is achieved, up to the recommended timing. Don't leave the color remover on an excessive amount of time. If it is necessary to do a second application, do so—only in the areas that are still too dark, using a stronger solution.

10. When the desired stage of lightening is achieved, rinse, shampoo, condition, and

towel dry the hair before the color application. Formulate, as always, mindful of the client's five key factors. If permanent haircoloring is used, 10 to 20 volume developer is often recommended, rather than extremely low volumes (the developer helps to even out any minor defects in the lightening). Demi-permanent haircoloring is frequently an excellent choice after decolorizing.

Sometimes Tint Does Lift Tint

There are exceptions to the rule about tint not lifting tint.

Many companies teach using a high-level color with a high-volume developer for spot lifting or very slight removal. This is a handy little technique when a color goes dark in an isolated area. Occasionally the temple area, hairline, or the tips of the hair will grab color, and rather than getting out the bleach, this is a very controlled and gentle way to quickly eliminate that unwanted deposit.

In addition, color clients often request highlights; you do not always have to highlight over color with bleach; high-lift tint is often sufficient to create the desired contrast.

Finally, one permanent haircoloring advertises that it is capable of removing some tint and coloring in the same step, within certain well-defined limitations. To an extent, all permanent color is capable of removing some tint, as in the case of using high-lift tint to highlight over a color or to do spot removal.

HAIR AFFECTED BY MINERALS

Minerals can be a problem in cities as well as in rural areas. Ground water or surface water, rural well water or city water—all can be hard. Certain geographical areas have particularly problematic water. If you have problem water,

Colorist's Clipboard

- Problem: Mineral build-up.

- Solution:
  1. Use a good demineralizing treatment and prescribe chelating shampoo.
  2. Any remaining off-cast caused by copper or iron may be concealed with a contrasting formula.

- Problem: Suspected medication build-up.

- Solution:
  1. Use a good clarifying or demineralizing treatment and prescribe clarifying shampoo.
  2. Use conditioning treatments as necessary.

you know it, and you have learned how to demineralize hair as much as possible. In regions where the local water is especially heavy with minerals, it may be routine to demineralize prior to almost all chemical services.

If you don't know whether or not you have a hard-water problem, then you do not; *you would know if you did*. The only thing you are apt to deal with is chlorine green (which is actually copper), or "swimmer's hair."

Chelating shampoos do reduce mineral deposits, and should be used by pool users and to prevent problematic build-ups in hard-water areas. Examples of **chelators** are **EDTA (ethylene diamine tetracetic acid)** and **DTPA (diethylene triamine pentaacetic acid)**. While the use of a chelating shampoo is good preventative technique, a chelating shampoo by itself is not nearly enough to remove a deposit of minerals that has developed over time and now presents an impediment to lightening or perming. Once the mineral has accumulated enough to be visible—to discolor the hair—or to interfere with chemical services, there is too much mineral for a shampoo alone to remove.

Build-ups of minerals, including swimming pool green, are removed with **demineralizing treatments** containing strong chelating ingredients. Numerous companies manufacture professional demineralizing treatments. Keep looking until you find one that works for you.

To eliminate discoloration caused by minerals, the first step is to treat the hair with a demineralizing treatment. An effective demineralizer will remove swimming pool green in most cases, and some iron-orange as well. Demineralize, and then color the hair as desired, using the principle of contrasting colors to conceal any remaining cast: blue to eliminate orange, red to contrast-out green,

red-orange for blue-green. The emphasis has to be on demineralizing, though. To effectively color over a mineral cast, the color must be deeper than the cast, which is in many cases as undesirable as the off-tone. Mineral deposits are usually not lifted satisfactorily, if at all, with tint or bleach.

Common Mineral Problems

Chlorine green (copper green), or swimmer's hair. Swimming pools are maintained with the addition of chlorine, primarily to kill bacteria, and also copper-containing algicides. Heaters can be a source of copper in pool water, too. The dissolved copper is deposited on whatever the pool water saturates. It is this copper which makes hair green (think of the green corrosion on copper pennies or pans). Copper plumbing in homes can also result in green hair.

On darker levels it may not be visible, but your comb, shears, and hands can detect chlorine damage even if you can't see a green cast. The hair feels stiff and coated, it is hardened and has a damaged feel and appearance, and it does not comb normally or cut normally. Pool water swells, pits, and abrades the cuticle.

Hair which has been permed, tinted, or bleached absorbs more copper than virgin hair. And hair that has been damaged by chlorine is more susceptible to damage from perm and color services.

Teach clients, especially chemical clients, how to prevent copper casts and minimize chlorine damage:

1. **Before you get into the pool, thoroughly saturate your hair with tap water (and you might also apply a pomade or heavy conditioner).**

Delores Davis

a colorist of long experience from Galax, Virginia, located in a mountainous region which is heavily mined and noted for its hard water:

"The effect of minerals is similar to metallic tint: more and more builds up until you can see it and feel it. Hydrogen peroxide tint applied over it is like tint over metallic salts, too—it may heat up or go dark very fast."

Dr. John Corbett

well-known cosmetic chemist and V.P. of Scientific and Technical affairs at one of the world's largest haircoloring companies:

"We are not aware of any effect that medications have on the haircoloring process. We have no real evidence that it does [have any effect]."

Sandie Talkington

stylist and owner of Accent on Styles in Stow, Ohio, has a somewhat different perspective:

"Every case is individual and has to be assessed individually . . .

"I don't assume it is okay to resume perming or coloring after chemotherapy or radiation, but I don't always say 'no,' either. That's why we have preliminary tests (patch tests and strand tests).

"The hair is much more porous after radiation—it is dried from the inside out.

"Chemotherapy weakens hair. If they don't lose their hair, I have continued coloring, but you have to use treatments more.

"I did this with my best friend—he was going through chemotherapy, he was 100 percent gray and he looked 100 years old without color. Not only was he sick but he looked it. It was important that he have color. He was on chemotherapy for a year and a half, which would have been even more miserable [without color]."

2. When you get out, don't wait—use a chelating shampoo right away. Don't sit in the sun or use a blow dryer when hair is wet with pool water.

Lime (magnesium and calcium). Lime is found in water almost everywhere. If there is excessive lime in your water supply, there will be a dull, whitish build-up on your shower tiles and shower doors. If you spray a window with the garden hose, the droplets will leave a flakey, whitish trace. Lime on hair dulls and hardens it, making it feel and look damaged.

Sulphur. Sulphur is also abundant in nature. It has a distinctive rotten-egg odor, so your nose tells you if there is a lot of it in your water. Sulphur is associated especially with the swamp water of lowlands, but it is found in many other places, as well.

Iron. Because iron colors the hair (and most everything else) you know if it is abundant in your water supply. Iron stains everything orange, wherever water drips, runs, or soaks: the porcelain in the bathroom and kitchen, the inside of the clothes washer, light-colored clothing, as well as hair which is light enough to show the stain. Light brown hair and lighter will pick up an orange cast. On darker levels, you can feel the build-up. Minerals make hair feel coarser, harder, almost brittle.

Sometimes you find out about an iron build-up only when you try to lighten the hair and the hair gets permanently stuck at the orange stage; that's not melanin—it's a mineral, which cannot be bleached out.

Homemade Demineralizers

Homemade remedies for mineral build-ups range from shampoo mixtures (peroxide shampoos, or shampoo with baking soda added), to lemon juice or vitamin C (ascorbic acid) mixed with distilled water and epsom salts. These mixtures effect some removal, but the most reliable and gentlest way to get minerals out of hair is with a product specifically made for that purpose. You don't want to damage her hair unnecessarily—the more porous you make it, the more vulnerable her hair will be when she gets back into the pool or shower.

HAIR AFFECTED BY MEDICATIONS

How do medications affect the haircoloring process? There are still more questions than answers on this subject, and often more speculation than information.

Some drugs do accumulate in the hair, but it does not automatically follow that these substances interfere with haircoloring or with any other salon process. Arsenic is the classic example of a substance taken internally that can be detected in hair. Arsenic is actually a metal, and metals have a great affinity for hair; lead poisoning, too, can be diagnosed via hair sampling. There are some drugs of abuse that can be detected in hair, cocaine especially. However, whether such uptakes have any impact on artificial haircoloring is another question entirely.

Changes in texture, condition, or color are sometimes observed in the hair of unwell clients. Some cancers can alter natural haircolor; hypothyroidism can make hair dry and lifeless; genetic or nutritional abnormalities (anemia or malnutrition, most notably) can cause changes in the texture and pigmentation of hair. So was it the medicine, or the illness, which affected your client's hair?

Certain medicines do affect the condition of hair, and even its pigmentation. Chemotherapy has a formidable impact on hair, because chemotherapy destroys fast growing cells, and hair is very fast growing; hair may be made very fragile or it may be lost, and hair regrown after loss to chemotherapy may be a different texture or color. There are rare instances of **hyperpigmentation** or **hypopigmentation** (darkening or graying) caused by medication; certain antimalarials are often cited. In these and a scant handful of other uncommon instances, medicine may alter the texture of hair, make it more fragile, or even change its color. But these are all exceptional cases, and their relevance to the question of whether or not medicine interferes with artificial haircoloring is unclear.

The essential question is: *Do medications affect hair enough, and in such a way, as to cause haircoloring formulas to fail?* At present there is no objective proof that medicines interfere with the haircoloring process, but it is not a question that has been answered definitively. It is probable that interference is minimal. We take lots of medicine in this country, and color our hair, too; the two do not appear to be incompatible. If drugs commonly interfered with haircoloring, given how much of them we consume, it would be hard to get color to perform with any consistency at all.

Although it is unlikely that any medicine the client is taking will make a difference in the haircoloring result, there is no harm in exercising caution and pretreating the hair with a **clarifying** or **detoxifying** product. Suspected cases of medication build-up are treated in the same way as mineral build-ups—with the use of demineralizing, purifying, or chelating treatments and shampoos. Despite the minimal chance of interference, this is good general technique.

Hair which is fragile, regardless of the cause, should be handled with great care and caution. Hair which is breaking should not be colored, or chemically treated in any way; it should be conditioned and made to appear as healthy as possible.

Cancer Patients—To Color or Not to Color?

What colorists do—what hairstylists do—is help clients look and feel better. With clients undergoing cancer treatment, looking and feeling better takes on a deeper meaning. The side effects can be overwhelming, and an extra measure of sensitivity and judgment is required of the colorist. Sometimes it may make sense to continue coloring; in other cases it may be wiser not to color.

"Look Good . . . Feel Better"

"Look Good . . . Feel Better" is a cooperative program of the American Cancer Society, the National Cosmetologists' Association, and the Cosmetics, Toiletries and Fragrance Association, the purpose of which is to help people through the physical changes of cancer and cancer therapy. Complimentary hair and make-up consultations are arranged for cancer patients and complimentary cosmetic kits supplied them. To learn how you can become involved, or to refer a cancer patient, call 1-800-395-LOOK.

Billie Capps

stylist and co-owner of Trendsetters Emporium in Warner Robins, Georgia, on coloring the hair of cancer patients:

"We don't recommend color during chemotherapy or radiation. There can be hair loss with both, and with chemotherapy, scalp changes—dryness or cracking, itching . . .

"Quite often it's not what the client wants to hear, and as colorists we want to do something for them. I usually will encourage them into a hairpiece if they want color change. I don't even do temporary color.

"We use hydrating products to keep the scalp as healthy as possible, and to relieve the dryness—nothing stimulating—you want to sedate as opposed to stimulate . . . I think it's a comfort factor."

partfive

5

marketing and management

The first chapter of this unit, Chapter Thirteen: Marketing and Promotion of Haircoloring Services, provides basic marketing background, discussion on some core marketing issues, specific promotional techniques, and ideas on how to talk to clients about color.

The last chapter, Chapter Fourteen: Other Helps and Tools, encompasses these topics: choosing color products, making the most of in-salon classes, client records, conversion to another color system, how to best use manufacturers' toll-free numbers (technical help lines), and recommended books, videos, organizations, and events.

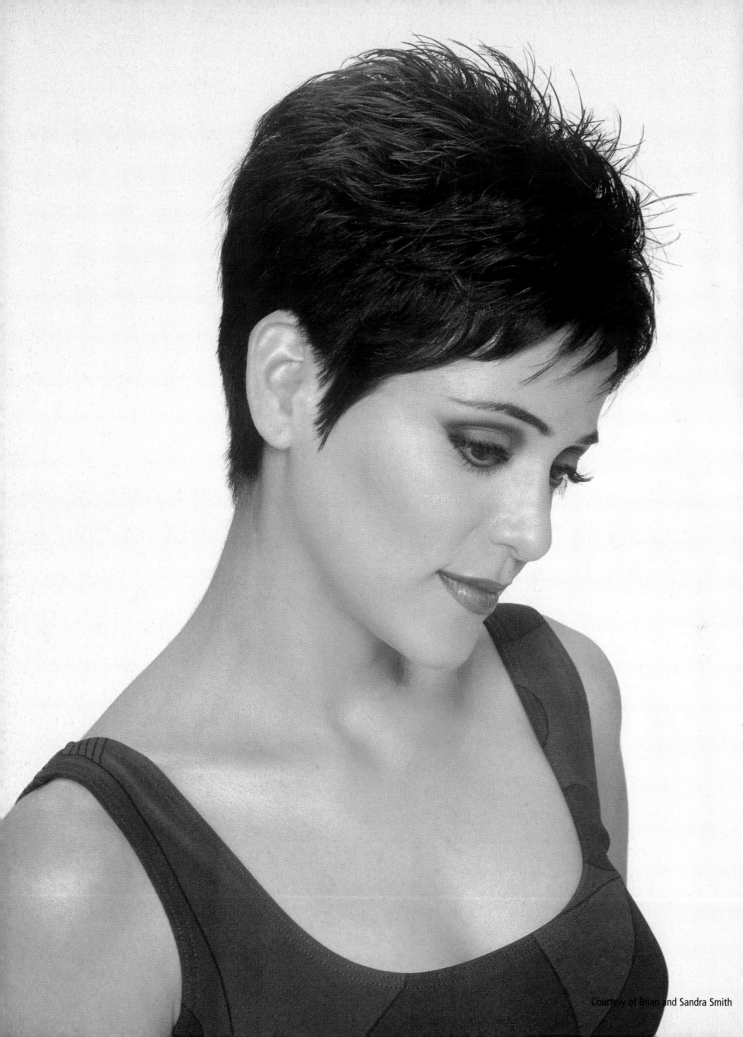

chapter thirteen

marketing and promotion of haircoloring services

Marketing is not the average stylist's favorite subject. (Is it yours?) Most of us would rather think about hair (or almost anything else). We would rather think about, talk about, and do hair, and let the rest of it take care of itself. Marketing? No thanks. Not only is it not very interesting, there is something intrinsically distasteful about it. It's calculating. It's manipulative. I don't want my clients to think I'm trying to sell them.

Marketing is more about planning your business, though, than it is about selling. Marketing is deciding what kind of business you are going to have, what you are going to provide your clients, and how you will do that and make a profit in the process. Most hairstylists are very client-focused, and that is really the essence of marketing. We do a lot of what is really "marketing" without being aware of it.

BASIC MARKETING ISSUES: YOUR CLIENTS AND WHAT THEY WANT

Marketing is not the same as selling. The sale (of a bottle of shampoo or a highlighting service) is the objective of marketing (and, at some level, it has to be your objective and mine—how else are we going to earn our pay?) but marketing is not selling. *Selling*, as a practice, is more about what the seller wants than what the buyer wants, it is seller-driven, whereas *marketing* is completely client-focused and client-driven. Marketing is all about understanding your clients' needs. You do not come to work to sell shampoo and highlightings; you come to help clients look and feel their very best. In a nutshell, **marketing** is the practice of identifying consumers' needs and meeting those needs, for a price.

Marketing answers these questions: Who, Where, What, When, and at What Price? Who do you want to serve—who is your target clientele, or **target market?** Where are these clients—where should you locate, and what kind of advertising will reach them? What services (and goods) do these clients want? When? (What should your hours be?) And what price do they want to pay?

Promotion is how you present your services and goods for sale—ways of calling attention to what it is you're selling. **Promoting** is creatively informing your clients (or potential clients) what it is you have for sale.

Much of marketing and promotion has to do with image-building ("**positioning**")—establishing in your clients' or potential clients' minds what kind of place your business is. What position in your clients' minds do you want to occupy? How do you want to be perceived? What reputation do you want? All your marketing and promotional efforts should be consistent with that imagery, that position.

But it all starts with deciding who your clients are. If your target market is upper-middle-class women and men, then your marketing and promotion have to zero in on them, and will be geared toward prestige and quality. You want an image consistent with (you want to position yourself on a par with) other fine businesses in your locale, such as fine clothing stores, a fine jewelry store, a prestigious interior design firm, fine eateries, and so forth.

Defining Your Target Market

Whom are you serving? Whom do you want to serve?

Who is your clientele currently, and is that the clientele you want to have?

Ideally, a business would have selected its target market way before it ever opened for business. Consider who is actually walking through the door to buy your services. If you have the type of clients you want, great. You probably want more. Maybe you want to try to get more of certain kinds of clients, and fewer of others.

What kinds of clients do you want to serve? Define your target market. Now think about what those clients really want from you.

You might ask clients, directly, what they want. On the client profile sheet that new clients fill out, ask, "Why did you leave your previous salon?" That's like asking, "What *don't* you want from a salon?" The answer reveals buying motives. Some salons have suggestion boxes, or do an occasional client survey. Bear in mind, though: not all suggestions are good suggestions, and sometimes clients fail to tell you what they really want. After defining your target clientele, defining what they want takes thoughtful consideration, and at least as much *good judgment* as inquiry.

Peter Drucker

business management expert and father of MBO (Management By Objectives):

"There will always, one can assume, be a need for some selling. But the aim of marketing is to make selling superfluous. The aim of marketing is to know and understand the customer so well that the product or service sells itself."

— *Drucker, P.F.,* Management: Tasks, Responsibilities, Practices *(New York, NY: Harper & Row, 1973) pp. 64–65.*

Designing Your Product

Your "product," as a salon or as an individual stylist, has two distinct aspects: first, what we broadly called "service," and second, the actual hairstyling services—color, cut, styling, or perm—that you perform.

Your clients expect a certain ambience and a certain level of customer service (or "guest service"). These intangibles are created by:

- **You—your conduct and appearance.**
- **The conduct and appearance of the salon staff (how the staff looks; how staff treat and talk to guests and to each other—dress, grooming, manners, attitude—what is commonly termed "professionalism"), which is a direct result of how employees are hired and trained.**
- **The atmosphere you create with location, storefront, decor, music, cleanliness, variety of services, and so on.**
- **The amenities you provide (choice of beverages, reading material, scalp massage at the shampoo bowl, and so forth).**
- **The imagery you create around your business through advertising, community involvement, professional achievements, and so forth.**

The sum total of all such details is the environment you create for your clientele, which is a big part of your product design and a big part of why clients come to you.

So: What kind of place do your clients want to come to and how do they want to be treated? Write it down to make it clear in your mind.

Colorist's Clipboard

Your target clientele and what they want:

- *What type of clients do you want to have?*

- *What do these clients expect from a salon?*

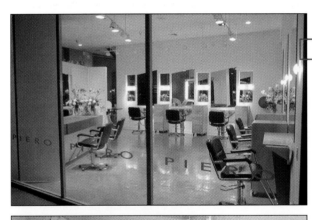

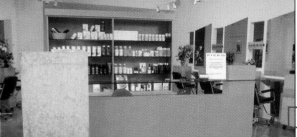

Courtesy of Piero Salon

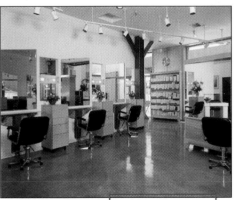

Courtesy of Piero Salon

Courtesy of Koger-LaPrairie for Salon JKL

Then, what services do your target clients need or want?

- **What actual haircoloring services do your clients need? (Gray coverage, gray blending, gray reduction, shading, brightening, and so on. What blonding services? Highlighting services? Reds?)**
- **How will you price these services?**
- **How will you prepare your staff to perform these services (recruitment and training methods)?**
- **How will you communicate these offerings to your clients (advertising, display, printed materials, promotions)?**

ESSENTIALS FOR SUCCESS

There is not one, pat marketing and management formula that works for every salon. Specific marketing strategies, promotional activities, compensation plans, training programs, managerial styles, and so forth differ among successful salons. What works for the salon across town, or for the person doing the seminar, may or may not apply to you: your clientele is not necessarily the same (your market may be different), you are not the same (you and your staff have different strengths, priorities, and personalities), and your salon may be larger or smaller, with relatively more or less overhead.

So specific tactics may very well differ, but there are at least two common threads in every success story. Regardless of size, price, or location, these two elements are unchanging in successful salons:

- **Clients are treated with courtesy.**
- **The salon does good work.**

People do business where they are treated with respect and consideration.

Customer Service: Courtesy, Comfort, and Cleanliness

Some salons believe in pampering, while others save their energy for doing hair. Maybe you serve fancy teas and treats, maybe you just put out a stack of styrofoam cups and turn on Mr. Coffee. Your client gowns may cost $50 apiece or $10 apiece. No matter how elaborate or simple the trappings, though, all people appreciate and even demand courtesy: a smile, "please," "thank you," a courteous greeting and farewell, a tissue if it's needed—the simple things. People do business where they are treated with respect and consideration.

Picture this: a circle of colorists at a color show, talking about tools and techniques to distinguish their work from color services available "just anywhere," and a salon owner says, "How about just being *kind?*"

That salon owner was Kenneth Anders, who has a highly successful business in the Columbus, Ohio area, Kenneth's Hair Designgroup. He was not dismissing the importance of professional tools and presentation ("showmanship," some say), just pointing out that there is no substitute for kindness. If the client doesn't feel like you care about her, nothing else you do matters. (There's an adage: Until people know how much you care, they don't care how much you know.)

"It used to be clients just came to us to look good," Kenneth says. "Now they come to us to look good and to feel good. How does the person feel during that service? Is their collar wet, is there color in their ears? Comfort is important."

If courtesy and comfort are the first rules of customer service, then cleanliness isn't far behind. A dirty, messy store makes you feel uneasy, unsure of the merchandise; you won't stay any longer than you have to and you may avoid going there in the future. Think about how a dirty bathroom makes you feel. What if the gown your doctor asked you to put on smelled like it hadn't been washed? Makes your skin crawl, doesn't it? We tend to take hair on the floor and color on the sink for granted, but to clients it is just unclean and unpleasant.

The Quality of Your Work

Word of mouth has always been—and still is—the best advertisement in the salon business. Every color you do is your best advertisement. If your work isn't good, you don't retain clients and you don't have clients to send you clients. Marketing can't make up for poor work.

What's good?

Most important, good haircoloring is becoming; it suits the client objectively and psychologically, it enhances her skin and eyes, and she feels good in it. Second, good haircoloring doesn't damage the hair unnecessarily; it leaves the hair healthy, or relatively healthy. Third, it's the right level(s) and tone(s), everywhere—front to back and scalp to ends. Fourth, it lasts as long as it's supposed to.

Beyond that, what's good is a matter of taste and timing. What you think is bad today you may like tomorrow. That's fashion. And what one person loves another may hate. That's personality and taste.

I once flipped through a Rolls-Royce brochure. Under engine size for one of the cars, it said "adequate." What is "adequate" for you? What is your standard of excellence?

THE ABCS OF PROMOTING SERVICES

"Promotions" are ways of making your services and products more known to clients or potential clients.

There are four main forms of promotional activity:

1. **Personal selling (professional recommendation).**
2. **Advertising and publicity (newspaper, radio, TV, direct mail).**
3. **In-salon sales promotions (displays, service menus, newsletters, other descriptive literature, service packages, gifts with purchase).**
4. **Presentations and other community involvement.**

Your **"promotional mix"** is how you blend these four forms of promotions.

Personal selling—your professional recommendation—is the most powerful and effective mechanism for the promotion of haircoloring services. (That word—*sell*—really *is* a four letter word, isn't it?!) I am not saying your professional recommendation is a sales pitch; it is not. You don't make the recommendation to make a sale; you recommend what you know will make the client look and feel great, because that is what stylists are supposed to do. That's our job. We sell through education; we inform clients; we give "beauty advice."

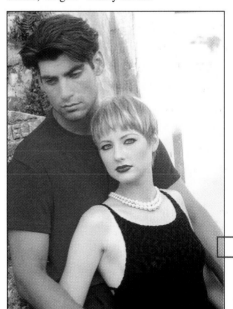

Courtesy of Koger-LaPrairie for Salon JKL

Michael Burton

salon owner and noted colorist of Michael Burton Colors, Atlanta, Georgia:

"I care more about people and less about money. I care about my work. I want to be the best haircolorist in the world—I won't ever be, but I want to be. It's my belief that if you do the best work, you'll make money. I only do six to eight clients a day . . . " (Then he walked me over to a client to show me an unusual color technique he had just done.) "I don't charge extra for this. It's not about how much extra you charge. It's about how much better your work is."

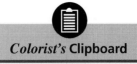
Personal selling does not cost anything. Presentations and community involvement don't have to cost anything but time. Publicity that you arrange, a press release that you write and send to the local paper before or after a community event, for instance, doesn't cost money, either. Manufacturers and distributors often provide free display items for in-salon advertising. The majority of promotions do not necessarily require a piece of your budget, but they do require time: thought, planning, effort, and follow-through.

The goals of promotional activity are:

1. **To put the salon name and your name before the public and build your professional image.**
2. **To encourage existing clients to buy more services and products.**
3. **To attract new clients.**

Promotions are goal directed. Promotional campaigns for color revolve around one central, underlying goal: building a reputation for haircoloring expertise. Specific themes might be: haircoloring trends; noncommitment haircoloring; fast, new techniques; natural, non-damaging color; men's color; personalized haircoloring; makeovers; or total beauty. It is less costly to promote business among existing clients than to increase your client base; selling more services and products to the clients you already have costs less than attracting new clients and selling to them.

Darleen Hakola calls her Portland, Oregon, salon "The Colour Authority." Her promotional theme is built right into the name of her business. "When we opened we knew what our image would be," she says. "It was going to be a color-with-cut salon."

HOW SALONS PROMOTE HAIRCOLORING SERVICES

Darleen Hakola, The Colour Authority, Portland, Oregon (12 stylists, 3 assistants). "You have to do good work and you have to tell people you do good work . . . reputation builds your salon.

"I all-the-time advertise in a local health and fitness book. There are seven or eight other periodicals that I advertise in, using the same ad in all of them because I've always been told repetition was important . . . You have to have a commitment to it if you are going to advertise."

Here's some copy from a few of Darleen's ads: "Let our team find the perfect haircut accented with a shiny haircolor just for you . . . Elle Magazine picks Darleen as a 'top colorist in the country' . . . Colour Authority predicts for fall: golden blonde, ravishing red, deep brunette . . . " Most prominent in all of the ads is her logo: the name of the salon, her name, and the words *Hair Colour Specialists*. Every ad has a large photo of great-looking hair.

If you call the Colour Authority and are put on hold, you don't hear music; you hear Darleen talking about the latest salon color services. A client of hers owns a company that makes on-hold tapes for businesses. Darleen writes the script, and the on-hold company makes the tape. She says it is "helpful, particularly in color, to identify the specialties that clients aren't aware of," such as gentle, deposit-only color, color glosses, and specialty techniques. Here's an excerpt from one of her on-hold tapes: "Ask for a free consultation and have haircolor better than the color you were born with . . . the Colour Authority is a member of the International Haircolor Exchange; this education qualifies us to be the best in our industry . . . "

Joe Santy, owner of Attitudes, Langhorne, Pennsylvania (7 stylists). "The biggest thing I do [to promote color] is one of the oldest; I use highlights to get clients used to color . . . three, four, five, half a dozen highlights . . . It takes you eight cents worth of bleach, six pieces of foil and eight minutes. I know I've never lost money doing that . . . I don't think discounting labor—direct mail coupons—is effective in creating loyal clients, but letting them experience it is."

Eric Fisher, Eric Fisher Salon, Witchita, Kansas (staff of 23). "Professional recommendation is basically how we promote color—'Let's break up the front with a few streaks'—and we use a 'look book.' " Eric puts styles and colors he likes into a binder, his "look book," to show clients. Every salon and every colorist can do this, using pictures from fashion magazines.

There is an emphasis on education at Eric's salon; there's always an educational event on the calendar. He brings in famous colorists to do workshops with his staff. Two evenings a week the salon has education as part of their assistantship training.

Steven Brooks, owner of Diva Studio and The Mens Room in Las Vegas, Nevada (12 stylists, 5 assistants). "We don't have a typical advertising campaign—we do zero advertising. I don't really believe in it so much. Maybe later on in our life cycle, to reinforce our image . . . " Steven and Lisa Brooks opened their salon in 1993, in an out-of-the-way office park with no walk-in traffic, a location that many owners would have considered disadvantageous. It was the building they

wanted, though, and they made the unusual location part of a hip, slightly off-beat image. "Nobody finds us without directions, and then they still get lost. So we turned it into our company motto," Steven says. " *'Do you know where Diva is?'* You might have heard of us, but have you ever found us?

"Color is 42 percent of our business and it's strictly word of mouth, because we do some killer color. That talks the loudest. When you've got a great cut and a great color, there isn't anything you can do that's better—yellow pages, radio, print—nothing is better than that. Just make sure you load her up with menus and business cards on the way out.

"We have a saying here: the good get gooder. [A clientele] grows exponentially, it isn't one client at a time. One client sends you four, those four send you 16 . . . Instead of dropping 500 dollars for a radio ad we use it on education, then it shows in our work . . . our clients are our walking advertisements."

Steven and Lisa also actively promote services. "We choose a corporation of the month and offer them half price on all services. We do [a professional hockey team] . . . We do service with service promotions—and we try to cross-mix services—free brow wax with cut, and then they're in the skin care department, too . . .

"We're on the Internet, worldwide. When you punch up "Diva Salon" you see a photo [of hair] . . . a description of the salon, a photo of the reception area, a list of the products we have." Steven talked about several recent clients that had found Diva through the Internet, among them a woman in Belgium who was coming to Las Vegas to get married and needed a stylist for her wedding day! (Their salon T-shirt has the salon logo on the front and the website on back!)

Colorist's Clipboard

There are four forms of promotions:

• *Professional recommendation.*

• *Advertising and publicity.*

• *In-salon advertising and promotions (displays, photos or posters of haircoloring, client color books, service packages, how your haircolor looks, and so forth).*

• *Presentations and community involvement.*

The goals of promotional activity are:

• *To build your reputation for excellence in haircoloring.*

• *To encourage existing clients who aren't "into" color to buy color services.*

• *To upgrade color services for clients who are "into" color.*

• *To attract new clients.*

Edie Noppenberger, Edie's Styling Center, Clearwater, Florida (3 stylists, 2 assistants). "There are a lot of ways to do marketing that don't cost a lot, for salons my size. Number one, I don't have ten thousand dollars for ads, and number two, I don't have the staff members to do it if they came in!

"I did a lot of creative marketing with a hospital, that for the most part I just had to pay printing . . . It takes energy and time but not a lot of money." The marketing director of a nearby hospital, a client of Edie's, facilitated her promotional efforts. (Every salon has among its clientele key personnel in local companies who are delighted to open doors for you!) "I did flyers that were put up on employee bulletin boards . . . sponsored the heart-a-thon walk [and distributed a card] for a discount on services—ten dollars off chemical services, valid for a limited period of time . . . and we did a makeover of hospital staff and fashion show with a local clothing store."

Albert and Susan Trombley, owners of Tromblay Salon and Gallery in Kalamazoo, Michigan (7 designers). Albert and Susan write a quarterly newsletter for their clients. It's upbeat, informative, not totally about hair (they've included stylist profiles, short articles on fashion, Susan's music picks) and it's very visual in design (creative use of fonts, layout, clipart, photos, color). This is some copy from an issue that zeroed in on color services:

"*Look deep into your eye*s (that's right—*your eyes*). See the tiny band of colors that ring your pupil? They're your personal color code—the palette you should choose from when considering a new hair hue. When a client asks for a new haircolor, we take careful inventory of the tones in his or her skin and eyes . . . We have proof that our results are gor-

geous: word-of-mouth referrals from happy clients have made haircoloring a big part of our business . . ."

Tromblay Salon is located in a renovated downtown building, with tall ceilings and big rooms, which means a lot of wall space. Albert and Susan found an almost-free way to fill their walls with art (and bring art lovers into their salon); they applied to make the salon an "alternative exhibition space" for the Kalamazoo Arts Council. A new exhibit is hung every other month, and the salon's only responsibility is to host an opening for the artist. No more bare walls and a great way to network with the community—not to mention the publicity. They get lots of print in Arts Council literature, regional tourism guides, and so forth. Here's how Tromblay is described: "This progressive, full-service salon is home to Kalamazoo's most unique gallery location . . . "!

John Hickox, owner of Hickox Salon and an advanced academy in Portland, Oregon (staff of 50). "We have a weekly downtown paper—an arts and entertainment weekly, not a trash magazine—that we advertise in. It's a lifestyle ad, meaning it isn't just a photo of a girl's head. It shows current clothing and current looks, with no copy. It'll be something we like, something the client can relate to but still a little on the edge.

"We're on TV about 20 or 30 times a year as 'the haircare experts,' and we've done that for ten years. We're considered regulars on a local morning talk show. We got on that show because we took care of all the news anchors . . . we developed credibilty with them. A couple weeks ago we turned models red, with the 'in' new haircut. That is a very visual, wonderful showcase for us.

"Twenty-two percent of our clients come from TV, and 72 percent come from referral. TV is nice to build an image, but the reality is most our customers come from people who send their friends. Only 5 percent is from advertising. But I think it is important that we continue to image to [clients] new fresh looks; they continually have to be stimulated. We have to keep them feeling confident that they're coming to the right place.

"Color is a big thing here; we love it, we believe in it. We constantly promote it to the client...there are a million reasons for people to wear color, all of them honest.

"We do overkill on training. We bring [name] educators into the salon for training . . . If anyone wants to come on board as a colorist they assist the head colorist and once a week have an academy day with live models. The head colorist has a written curriculum that looks like a phone book."

Mark Foley, marketing consultant and owner of Lockworks Hair Image in Calgary, Alberta, Canada. Mark suggests designing a service menu with brief descriptions of color services, in language clients can relate to. He recommends that the salon owner create a variety of color services that specifically appeal to different types of clients, giving each a unique name and a short description. "Step back and look at those services from the client's point of view. The very same permanent haircoloring can be called one thing for the mature male market, another for the

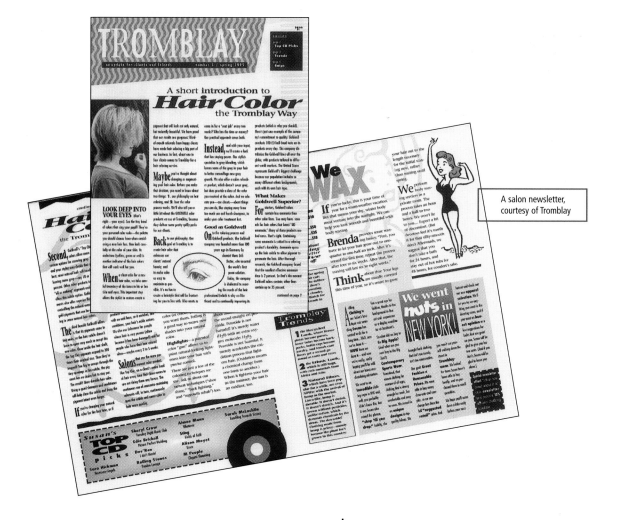

A salon newsletter, courtesy of Tromblay

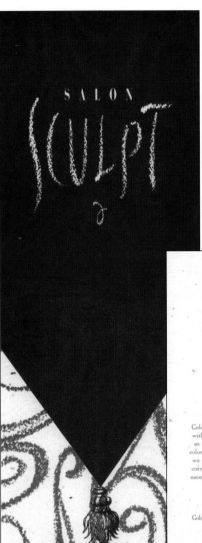

younger male market, for the mature female market, the career woman, the fashion-oriented, the youth market—and the same with all other kinds of color services . . . Some hair designers are good salespeople, some aren't. The reason for having a menu like this is to communicate your offerings even if the designer doesn't."

For instance: the blending technique that you use for graying men? Give it a name (naturalizing, color blend) and write a sentence or two about how it looks (natural, subtle, years younger, masculine, executive appeal, image update for gentlemen); call the same blending technique something else for women and describe it in terms meaningful to women.

Don and Flonnie Westbrook, owners of Elon Salon, Marietta, Georgia (11 stylists, 10 apprentices). This salon runs newspaper ads that don't look like ads at all, but more like articles (journalists call these "advertorials" or "info-ads"). The "headline" of the ad will say something like "The Return to Glamour" or "Fall into Color" (a September theme). Each ad has two or three great-looking photos of hair, and a fashion story focusing on trends in haircoloring. Toward the end of the "article" there will be a paragraph or two about the salon, or about Don and Flonnie themselves ("With their expertise and knowledge, Don and Flonnie have pushed to the forefront of the hair industry to become the leading edge authorities in haircolor . . .").

Robert Austin Miller, owner of Antoine Du Chez Hair Salons and Day Spas (four locations) and a cosmetology school in Denver, Colorado (totaling around 200 employees). "The promotion of haircoloring plays a big part in schools, too, in that color is where the money is made in the industry today.

"In most schools and salons people direct their marketing toward the young, the advant-garde—what you call a 'niche market'—we market for the baby boomer up, because they are more likely to color their hair . . . that's your bread and butter, the person with the 37K income and two kids . . . as artists we like to explore the extremes, but that's not where the money is.

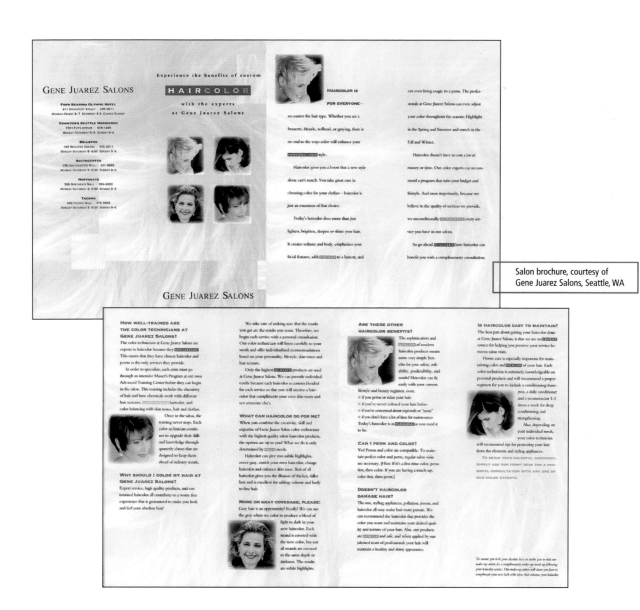

Salon brochure, courtesy of
Gene Juarez Salons, Seattle, WA

"[We promote haircoloring] by the color we do . . . the visual of it is really the marketing piece. If it's good they tell two, three, four people—if something's not right they tell 12 people . . . We research our data base by who has not had color, and do a direct marketing piece to them . . . We do introductory promotions—with the haircut you receive a demi color for free, brighten up your hair for summer. Eighty percent of the time they stay with it. Transfer that to permanent color and you have a client forever."

Roy Peters, Dallas, Texas, famous haircoloring educator. Roy accidentally discovered a great promotional technique early on in his career. As a new stylist, he collected hair clippings and colored them to learn about haircoloring. One day he was showing some of his practice swatches to a client, and she said, "I like that one. What would my hair look like with that color?"

Roy replied, "That *is* your hair"—it was a clipping from her last cut—and of course that

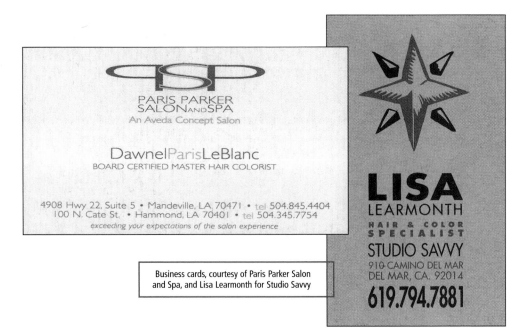

Business cards, courtesy of Paris Parker Salon
and Spa, and Lisa Learmonth for Studio Savvy

was the day he started coloring her. He had dis-covered he could use his practice swatches to promote color services!

Whenever you cut an inch and a half or more, keep some of the hair. Do a variety of colors for each client, and tape the mini-swatches on a card labelled with the client's name. Show off the results at the next visit. Roy says that clients are so pleased and impressed that you would make such an effort for them, they almost feel obligated to have a color service!

Donna Jean Tenbrink, esteemed cosme-tologist and cosmetology instructor, Gales-burg, Michigan. Donna Jean teaches stylists to promote services and loyalty by always hav-ing a plan for clients. Give clients a program of care: what she should do with her hair between this visit and the next, what the next visit will entail, and something a little different she might try a few months up the road. Show clients you are thinking up ideas for them by returning from a hair show with a new idea just for her, or by showing her a picture from a magazine that you saved because it resembles a color you would like her to try.

Robert Oppenhiem, author of *101 Promotional Ideas* (Milady Publishing Co.). Robert calls one particular promotional idea "the daddy of them all"—and it's something so simple it's easy to overlook. "Every living human being in the salon should have their hair colored," he says. It sounds obvious,"—and yet you would be surprised at the mousy browns, the gray roots . . .

"There are a million promotions, but the most important thing is for clients to have total confidence in your expertise. Number one, people should look at you and say, 'If I could have my hair colored to look like that, I'd have it done in a minute!' I don't care if it's a two-operator salon or a 20-operator salon. Stylists should come in on a Sunday or a Monday and color their hair—and if possi-ble everyone should get a color different from the one they already had—a color and a style—do makeovers on themselves.

"What keeps women from tinting their hair is fear . . . all the horrible tint they've seen. But when they come in and they look around and everyone has gorgeous color—healthy, decently styled, and all different—*that's* a color promotion!"

STYLIST TRAINING—NECESSARY TO ANY MARKETING PROGRAM

In the hairstyling business, what we sell is skill; we sell our ability to make clients look and feel better. Without skill, there is nothing to market. A salon cannot advertise haircoloring expertise and then be unprepared when the clients come in. And we can't ever stop becoming more skillful, or the clients move on. We can't be static because client needs are not static.

Listen to Bruce du Bois, Director of Education at Pierre & Carlo in Philadelphia, Pennsylvania: "I think sometimes we overdo it in terms of marketing color to clients . . . It may be more important to market color internally, to the colorists—to give the colorists good education on how to approach their clients artistically—making a beautiful picture come true rather than simply satisfying a need like 'cover my gray' or 'make my highlights ash.' "

Colorist's Clipboard

More ways to promote:

• *Rewrite your service menu to reflect the great variety of color services you do, using language clients understand.*

• *Write and mail a quarterly or twice-yearly newsletter to clients to inform them about haircoloring options and your expertise.*

• *Mail a postcard to salon clients that you aren't yet coloring, offering a complimentary consultation and half-off on a color service.*

• *Utilize display or promotional items that color manufacturers provide (client books, counter signs, and so forth).*

• *Clients want to help you be successful. What companies can your clients help you do promotions with? What special skills do clients have that might help you promote business?*

• *Get on TV, radio, the Internet, newspapers, magazines. Talk about and show your work, via community interest articles, beauty columns, paid advertising, press releases, and so forth.*

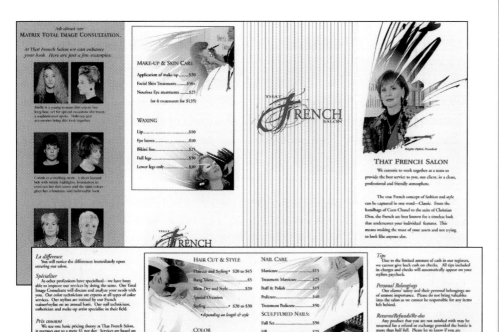

Salon brochure, courtesy of That French Salon

The color company whose products you use should be a steady source of education. Jerry Gordon, owner, J. Gordon Designs Ltd., Chicago, Illinois, puts it this way: "The first and foremost thing in marketing is having an affiliation with a manufacturer. You can't market anything you don't know. You need to know everything about the line and how it works. In the beauty business, that's how you market . . . If a company offers courses, take every single course."

Manufacturers' classes are essential, but not the sum total of salon training. Many salons also put together their own educational events, with staff members or guest colorists officiating.

LeeAnn Nelbach, owner of The Kindest Cut in Springfield, Virginia, names three staff members to a salon haircoloring team (the salan also has a cutting team, a perming team, and a long hairdressing team). "Each team is responsible for going out and learning about new techniques, learning new vocabulary [associated with services] . . . and making sure the staff gets the information. [Teams get their information from] hair shows, magazines, and schooling. One team does a hands-on or product knowledge demo at each staff meeting. We have a two-hour meeting once a month, one hour of which is devoted to the demo of a particular team. Not only does it keep the staff informed, but it also keeps them involved and working together."

Every six months, Belinda and Frank Gambuzza's Salon Visage in Knoxville, Tennessee, has a training event they call a "soiree." It is a self-made hair show in which all the salon employees participate. Two months before the soiree, staff members start working on looks they will present. Cutters look for trends in shape and texture; colorists look for what's happening in color; nail and make-up artists research trends in their specialities. Then they team up, select models, and plan total looks. The day of the soiree, models are cut and colored, their make-up and nails are done, they're dressed fashionably, and then, that evening, all the models are presented to the entire staff. Belinda and Frank assist, but the ideas and the work are the designers' own.

Frank explains the reason for the soiree: "After that night, there is a story to tell—'curly hair is coming back, color is getting bolder.' Everybody is on the same page, they are saying the same thing; that's the only way you can work together as a team."

"What you are doing is giving them ammuniation to help their clients," Belinda says. "When somebody comes in and says, 'What's new? What can I do?'—[the designers] think back to the soiree and say, 'Here's what's happening.' I could sit here all day long and say 'Why aren't you guys telling people about new trends [and services], why aren't you doing this'—well, how can they, if they don't have the information?"

DEPARTMENTALIZATION AND SPECIALIZATION

Departmentalizing means designating an area of the salon for haircoloring and an area for cutting. Departmentalized salons often have **specialized** stylists—cutters cut (and usually also perm) and colorists color—just as nail services and skin care have long been treated as distinct specialties. Cutter and colorist work together to achieve the final look; they consult and collaborate, but do not direct each other.

Approaches and Opinions Vary

Leland Hirsch says of his New York City salon, "Nubest opened in 1973 as a departmentalized salon . . . salons should be planned and decorated to be more specialized. If not a color department, then a daylight space to do color . . ."

Hickox Salon in Portland, Oregon, is "mostly departmentalized," says owner John Hickox. "We've done it both ways, it works both ways. But I like a color department because they're doing color all the time; I think their skill level remains higher. [We have a] color specialist team of four people and that's all they do."

At The Peller Salon in Atlanta, Georgia, there are eight stylists, two assistants, and one full-time colorist. Jason Peller says, "I like the idea of departmentalizing. You are using your skills to the utmost. It has been said many times that the jack of all trades is the master of none . . . We have a salon colorist; she does all my color, and the other stylists are learning to have her do their color. We are all the time talking about what color will work with the cut. The client feels like, 'Hey—I've got two people that *really like* what I'm going to look like—this is great!' "

Belinda and Frank Gambuzza, owners of Salon Visage in Knoxville, Tennessee, believe strongly in the value of specialization. "What happened [when we specialized] was exactly what we were told," says Belinda. "We had growth by at least forty to fifty percent. Because, if you think about specialization, you are using every chair in your salon [all the time] . . . It has been a tremendous growth process for us, and it has set us apart from anybody else in the city." A year and a half after specializing they opened a second salon, and now have three locations.

The Panopoulos Salons in Grand Rapids, Michigan, have color *areas* or color rooms, but not color departments. Max Matteson, CEO of Salon Enterprises (a salon group that includes the Panopoulos Salons, nine locations, and Haircuts Plus salons with 14 locations, as well as three cosmetology schools), explains their approach: "In our company we don't believe in the color department as such. We don't have colorists who just color hair. They might oversee those services, but we don't take the opportunity away from the haircutter to do color. I don't like it from an artistic point of view—the stylist should have all the tools to create a total image . . . and I don't like it from a business point of view . . . I don't want four or five prima donnas [controlling the salon's color business]." Then he talks about the color rooms: "You need to focus on haircolor if you're going to market it. If you have a color room it should say, 'Color Room'! There should be visual cues that color is done there—color products, swatches, posters, the right lighting for color . . ."

Kenneth Anders' salons, the Kenneth Hair Designgroup in Columbus, Ohio, are not specialized either. He says, "How can I take that away from my stylists? Forty or 60 percent of their income is color."

Reginald Laws, owner of PR&Partners Salons in the Washington, D.C. area, agrees: "I don't think it's important to have a department. It's important to have a philosophy. You are the color department. You can put a sign over your head if you want to, but it's your attitude that makes the difference."

I've Decided to Departmentalize and Specialize; How Do I Go About It?

Frank and Belinda Gambuzza made the transition to departments in 1991, when it was a very new, even unknown, concept in Knoxville. Belinda says they were apprehensive

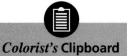

Colorist's Clipboard

Departmentalization and specialization

• *Specialization means that some stylists only cut, some only do color. Departmentalization means haircoloring is done in one area of the salon, cutting in another.*

• *A salon staff may be partly or fully specialized.*

• *Whether specializing or departmentalizing is right for your salon depends on your marketplace, your goals, and how much momentum you have in your current way of operating.*

• *Even if staff does not specialize, a salon can become more specialized in color by increasing training, improving lighting, adding color processing equipment, and so on.*

The language of color

• *Ways to open a consultation:*

  "What can we do for you today?"

  "What are you thinking about your hair?"

• *Ways to move from what she is thinking, to what you are thinking, without appearing to disagree with her:*

  "You know what I think would look really good?"

  "Another great option for you is . . . "

• *Ways to interest a client who hasn't expressed any interest in color:*

  "What are your plans for color?"

  "I have an idea, for later. Would you like to hear it?"

• *If you think the time is right, tell her about a variation on her color that she might enjoy at a future time and make a note of it on her client card.*

• *How you describe an idea can make all the difference in how people respond; consider how appealing your words are, but be specific, as well.*

about it, but they decided "even if it meant starting over, it would still be the best thing for us."

First, they departmentalized their building, adding a color room. "Everybody was still doing everything," Belinda explains. "If you were doing a haircut, you were in one area and if you were doing a color you were doing it in the color area, so they were going back and forth—and at first it was kind of crazy, but we were getting everybody into the mode of being in a certain department doing a certain thing. Then we started talking about total specialization."

The next step was to gradually departmentalize the staff, a process that took eight or nine months to complete. Frank and Belinda were the first to specialize, he in cutting and she in color. Each month two more employees made the change. "We talked to each one of our staff members, as individuals and as a group, and asked them what they would be interested in. They were all scared to death, just as we were! But as we did it, each staff member kept on saying, 'Oh my gosh! This is the best thing that ever happened to me! I just love it, I love being focused in on one thing'—so the people who were waiting to change couldn't *wait* to change.

"We put out a letter to all of our clients, defining what specialization is. For every one client we lost, there were two calling up saying 'I hear you specialize, I think that's great!' Even the clients that were a little upset at first have all eventually come back. It has been a tremendous growth process for us."

When the Gambuzzas made the decision to specialize, they had one salon and 20 employees. Five years later, they had two salons and 75 employees, ten of them full-time colorists, and were planning a third salon.

THE LANGUAGE OF COLOR (RECOMMENDING AND TALKING COLOR)

Most stylists agree: The consultation is the most important part of the appointment. It's when you gain the client's trust and plan the color service. Most agree, too, that the best consultations are brief and to the point—stretch it out too much and you may confuse both the client and yourself.

Consultation Basics

Clay Wilson of Doyle Wilson Salon, Los Angeles, California, teaches stylists to first listen, then recommend. "We'll begin by asking what we can do for them that day, and listen to everything they have to say. Then we'll say, 'You know what I think would look really good?' or 'Another option would be—.' And it's important to give them change, have a future for them—'and you know what we'll do later?'—work from solid colors into highlights, and seasonal changes . . . their hair should always be a work in progress."

You will find more information on the consultation process in Chapter Five: Communicating with the Client (pages 53–60).

Talking to Clients Who Have Not Yet Expressed Interest in Color

Jerry Poer, owner of a salon (Charleston, Charleston!) and school (Charleston Cosmetology Institute) in Charleston, South Carolina, gets clients thinking about color by asking, "What are your plans for color?" This approach puts the ball in the client's court; she doesn't feel like she's being "sold." If she hasn't thought much about color, now she's thinking about it, and she will reply, "I don't know; what do you think?"

Don Westbrook of Elon Salon, Marietta, Georgia, shared the following tip at a seminar. When he gets a client who is not yet into color, he says: "I have an idea, for later. Would you like to hear it?" No one ever said "no" to that; everybody wants to hear about themselves, and because it's "for later" the pressure is off—you aren't asking her to make an immediate decision. (Of course, if she likes the idea, Don usually has somebody available to do the service right away.)

These, then, are two direct-but-tactful ways to spur interest in color—professional all the way:

1. **"What are your plans for color?"**
2. **"I have an idea, for later. Would you like to hear it?"**

When the Color Is Finished
And once the color is complete?

Some stylists tend to be highly critical of their own work and have to be careful not to plant dissatisfaction in clients' minds—not that truly unacceptable results should go uncorrected. If there is a problem with a color result, it must be acknowledged and fixed, but it is unproductive to point out minor imperfections that the average person would not even notice. Do make a note on the client card if you think you should do something differently next time, and also note any additional services or options you discussed with the client.

Appealing Language

Charles Gregory of the Charles Gregory Salon in Atlanta, Georgia, offers a color service called "carmelizing." Sounds luscious, doesn't it? Phrases like "tortoiseshelling," "color glazing," and "gray marbleizing" appeal to people; they sound intriguing and get people's attention.

Language like this is also vague, however. Specific words, or pictures, swatches, and other visuals, have to be used, too, to make sure you and the client understand each other. Too many vague superlatives and there's no telling *what* the client really expects.

Appealing Words

Blonds: delicate, luminous, sunny, honey, amber, beige, wheat, caramel, ginger	Add dimension, texture, contrast, interest
Reds: deep, soft, subtle; fiery, vivid, hot; redwood, vermilion, copper, apricot, cinnamon	Feminine, masculine
	Younger, takes years off
Browns: rich, with dimension, shimmery, glowy, chocolate, chestnut, bronze.	Beautiful, exquisite, elegant, radiant, refined, sophisticated
Hues, tones, undertone, top tone	Gentle, nondamaging
Nuance, blend, soft	Noncommittal color, nonammonia, no peroxide, won't turn red
Translucent	Becoming, complimentary, suitable, what I see for you
Natural, healthy	
Bold, bright, intense, strong	Individualized, personal look, personalized, accentuate your natural coloring, customized
Gloss, shine, sparkle, sunlit, shimmery	

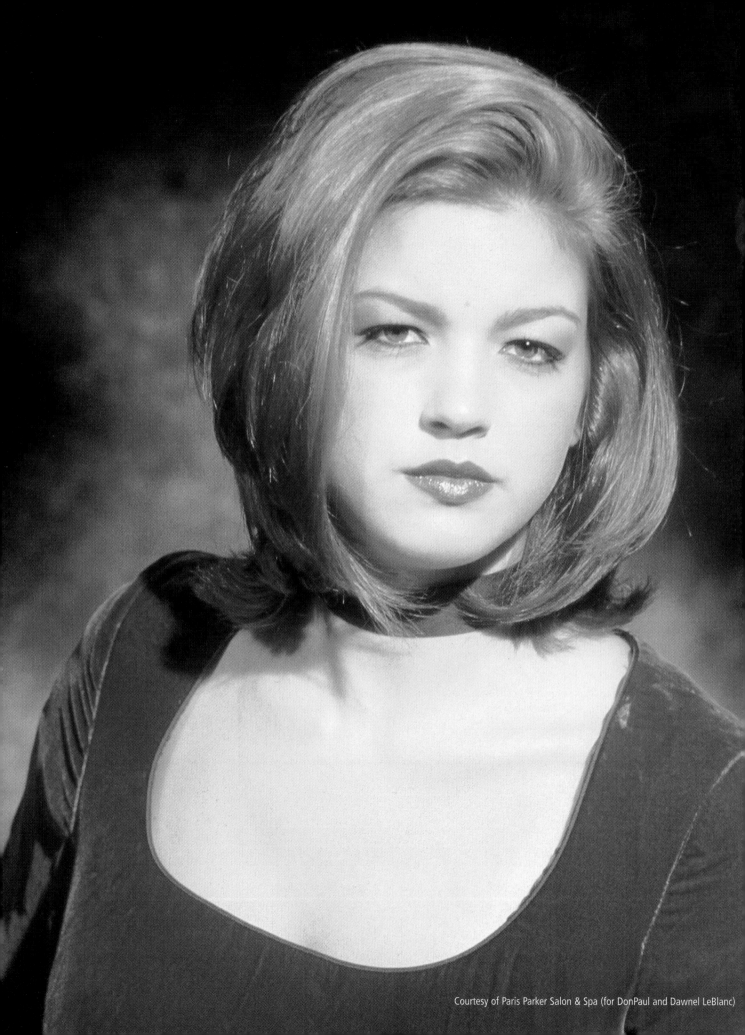

Courtesy of Paris Parker Salon & Spa (for DonPaul and Dawnel LeBlanc)

other help and tools

There is more to a color business than coloring hair. Business has us always making decisions, looking for information, negotiating change. This chapter deals with a few of the details of management that are critical to the day-to-day operation of a color business: choosing and changing products, planning classes, keeping records, and locating and utilizing outside resources.

SELECTING HAIRCOLORING PRODUCTS KNOWLEDGEABLY

If you go in search of the perfect color product, you will be disappointed over and over again. There isn't one. If there was a perfect product, one color would be all we would need, *only* that one would exist, and we would all be using it!

Shopping for a haircoloring product is like selecting a mate: You look for one with the attributes you most desire, and with flaws you can live with—like people, haircoloring products are never perfect. All do certain things very well (there are outstanding things about every product) and all are somehow flawed. (Some are more flawed than others!) That's the nature of the beast.

No one color product does all things better than all other products. Every color has special attributes, virtues, and shortcomings. To be—in all ways—the best, would be impossible. You cannot ask a shampoo to condition as well as it cleans; it is impossible. How can a color cover gray opaquely and be translucent, too?

A very drab base pigmentation that makes your blonds so neutral may prevent you from achieving strong golds. And the reds may be gorgeous, but not quite what you are looking for or accustomed to. (Red haircoloring is sort of like red lipstick—there is an endless array of red tones just a tiny bit different from each another.) No product can be all things to all people.

A good colorist can formulate a good product to compensate for its shortcomings, and to maximize its strengths.

Choose the product, or products, that you can work with the best, the one(s) you like the best. Make sure you use only professional goods. Choose a company, or companies, that you can respect and rely on—companies that respect *you*.

The products you use have to be cost effective for your salon. The manufacturer should offer high-quality in-salon classes. The sales representative should give you good service. You should have a good general level of satisfaction with the company's literature, toll-free help line, education, and so forth. And the company's philosophy and way of doing business should harmonize with your own.

Consider what color services you want to offer. What products do you need to carry out those services? Your products are your tools. Are you getting the lift, the tones, the wear, the coverage, the conditioning, and the pricing you have to have? Trade magazines and shows help you keep up with products; you have to know what's out there to select what's best for your salon.

"The Best of the Best"

Stacie Sanderford is a respected and immensely talented colorist who works at Diva Studio in Las Vegas, Nevada (owned by Lisa and Steven Brooks). The salon has a "best-of-the-best" rack in the retail area (shelves devoted to outstanding items from various retail lines). Stacie suggested they do the same with color products: pick out especially effective or one-of-a-kind items from a variety of color systems and use these to augment their main color line.

For instance: If your main color line doesn't have a beige series, you might stock the beiges from another system. Maybe your color line doesn't have reds quite the tone you want for certain clients; you might take three or four reds from another system to supplement those of your main line. There are outstanding items in every color system. Although you can't have every color product every staff member likes, borrowing from several different lines can be a practical way to create a high-performance dispensary.

Jerry Gordon

Chicago, Illinois, has been a hairdresser for 40 years and a salon owner for 22. He says this about selecting a color line:

"My decisions are based on what [the manufacturer] can do for me. If I don't get some payback for using the product over a period of years—training for my employees, publicity—I'm going to look for another product . . . Your staff gets bored. If you don't have a manufacturer to help keep up the interest level in the salon—constant training is the biggest thing—then, they don't want to bother with you; why bother with them? I want somebody who's going to work with me."

CONVERSION TO A NEW COLOR SYSTEM

Here are a few pointers to smooth the transition from one haircoloring system to another.

Set aside the old. If you are not just adding to what you carry but are eliminating the previous color product from your dispensary, then immerse the salon in the new and completely set aside the old. Hanging onto the old will only cause confusion.

All previous color experience serves in the use of another product, and most of what you did in the past will apply to the new product. But expect differences. There are some things about your past color use that literally will have to be forgotten. Where the new system differs from the old, forget what you used to do. Developer usage and ratios may differ. The level system may differ. Tones will be different. Don't balk at the change; train yourself to the new and lay the old to rest. You want the new color line to be as second nature to you as the previous one was.

Read all the information the manufacturer provides. Anything a manufacturer puts into print is highly reliable. The manual, fact sheets, package inserts—read it all. Color companies want you to be successful with their products; they do not write things that will detract from your success. In fact, literature is painstakingly engineered to increase your success.

Sometimes the manufacturer's directions are the course of last resort in a salon: unread until a problem arises. Let it not be so in your salon. Reading the literature is one of the simplest and best ways to work smarter.

The late, one-of-a-kind Arnie Miller, founder of one of the world's largest professional color companies and himself a hairdresser, used to say this about manufacturer's

directions: "We should stamp them, *'Top secret! Confidential! Do not read!'* Then *everybody* would read them!"

Schedule a product knowledge class. The best time for an introductory product knowledge class is shortly after you have gotten the product into the salon—two weeks, say. The system is totally set up in the dispensary, all the staff has read the literature, and you have had a chance to do some color with it. (Some familiarity with the new product will make what the educator says more meaningful.)

Don't hesitate to use the manufacturer's toll-free professional or technical help line. If you can't find an answer in the manufacturer's literature, or if you have any doubt about how to proceed, don't ever hesitate to call the color company! If you have three questions in one day, call three times! That's why they have a toll-free number.

While you are on the phone, tell the hot line consultant what printed materials you have and ask her if there is anything else available; your sales consultant may not have access to all available literature.

Reeducate your eye to the new system. Interpretation of levels is likely to differ in a new color system. Do not continue talking and thinking the old level system. You will confuse yourself and the people around you. If the line you are now using interprets levels differently, then you must interpret levels differently. The level system you are using is the only one that matters. Tones will be different, too. Unlearn the old.

The best way to reeducate your eye and your mind is to study the manufacturer's swatches. Get yourself in a quiet place, preferably alone, when you have 20 minutes to devote to the following exercise.

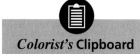

Colorist's **Clipboard**

Selecting color products

- *Does the color perform? Does it give you the tones, levels, conditioning, and coverage you need?*

- *What educational support does the company offer? Marketing support? How's the service and pricing?*

**Haircoloring products
are not identical.**

Colorist's **Clipboard**

Conversion to a new
color system

• *Read all manufacturer's
directions.*

• *Call the color company's
toll-free help line whenever
questions arise.*

• *Have a basic product
knowledge class.*

• *Reeducate your eye to the
new system.*

• *Try all the tones and techniques in the new system.*

• *Use comparison charts
advisedly.*

• *Formulate simply and learn
from every color you do.*

• *Plan some promotional activity around the new product.*

1. **Get the swatch chart out. Don't use a paper chart; level and tone on paper are never accurate.**
2. **Start with the neutral (natural) series swatches. Sweep your eyes up and down the series.**
3. **Read each level number and name in the neutral series aloud, from #1 on up, glancing at the corresponding swatch. Say aloud, "#1, black; #2, brown-black," and so on.**
4. **Now: Examine each of the neutral series swatches intently, one at a time, as though you had never seen them before and will never see them again! Try to memorize the way each level looks. Notice how different #1 is from #2, #2 is from #3, #3 from #4. Say the number and name of each neutral series swatch aloud again, as you concentrate for a few seconds on each. (Where do the colors "break" from light brown to dark blond? Is it 5 into 6? 6 into 7? Memorize this breaking point; it will help you keep all the numbers straight.)**
5. **Now look carefully at the tone of the neutral series. Does it look natural to you? Which of your clients will prefer this series?**
6. **Then you are ready to study another tonal series. Look at the gold swatches. Sweep your eyes over the series, noticing the graduation of depth to lightness. Is it consistent with the neutral series? Read aloud the number**
and name of each swatch in the series, from deepest to lightest, concentrating for a second on each. And what about the tone of the gold series—how gold is it? Do you like it? Are these wearable, pretty colors? Which of your clients can you visualize in these?
7. **Then study whatever series remain, in the same manner.**

This exercise is a sure-fire way to familiarize yourself with a new color system (or an old one that still seems awkward). Try it!

Try every product, tonal series, and technique in your new system. Don't get stuck in a rut and use only certain parts of your color system. If there is more than one color product in the dispensary, use them all. Use all of the tonal series in each. It is easy to get hung up on certain products or tones and ignore the others, but there is a purpose and a need for every bottle or tube on the dispensary shelves.

If the manufacturer recommends more than one way of filling, blonding, or covering gray, then try all the recommended techniques. Until you try something yourself, you can't form an opinion about it.

Use comparison charts advisedly. Comparison charts provide only estimates. If manufacturers' color systems were all identical, then comparison charts would be perfectly accurate; they are not, haircoloring products are not identical. Therefore, there are not perfect matches in every color line for every other color line. Comparison charts can provide only estimates—hopefully, close estimates. It is a mistake to convert clients from one color line to another simply by referring to a comparison chart.

A conversion should be handled like a first-time color consultation, using the swatches of the new system to identify the level and tone of the color you want to duplicate. The formula will be more accurate and the result more satisfactory if you formulate as you normally would (as you would at any other time for any other client for whom you are writing a formula), using the Universal Method.

If you want to use a comparison chart, the time to do so is after you have written the formula, to see if it is similar to what the chart says. This is a way of double-checking your work. It is not necessary, but confirmation of this kind can help you feel more confident when you are doing conversions.

Plan a launch! The introduction of a new product is an opportunity to do some promotional activity. Whether it is a new color glossing service you will offer, a colored shampoo, four new reds, or a whole new color system, plan a promotion of some kind around it, put it in the spotlight. ("Promotion" does not necessarily mean a price promotion—it may involve display, stylist incentive, a splashy mailer, and so on. Your color company or sales consultant can help you with promotional ideas.)

USING A COLOR COMPANY'S TOLL-FREE NUMBER

The toll-free number (professional line, technical line, hot line, help line) can be an invaluable resource. Here are some tips to help you use it to your best advantage.

Come to the phone prepared. Do not call the help line number until you have properly analyzed the client's hair and pinpointed the desired end result. Be sure the hot line expert knows the client's key factors (natural base level, percentage of gray, texture, porosity,

existing tint), and the exact level and tone that you want to create.

You cannot expect a good answer if you do not provide accurate and complete information. Remember: the person at the other end of the phone can't see the hair. They are relying on what you tell them.

Bring the swatch book(s) to the phone to help you communicate with the consultant, and bring pencil and paper to write down her recommendations.

Consider the product expert your colleague and call for her opinion whenever you are uncertain. The ideal time to call the help line is before you mix color—after the consultation, and before mixing. What you are doing is requesting a second opinion. Rather than considering the hot line your contingency plan, what you will do if all else fails, turn to it first, whenever you are uncertain.

Your client doesn't have to know that you are seeking another opinion, but if you must tell her, she will know she can count on you to get answers if you don't have all the answers, and she will know that you care more about her hair than your ego. This is no different than the doctor who calls a colleague into the examining room before deciding on a course of care.

If you are still uncertain when you get off the phone, do a preliminary strand test. Apply the suggested formula to an inch- or half-inch-square strand and see how it does. If it isn't what you want, call the hot line back and ask how to adjust the formula.

The manufacturer's hot line is not just a crisis number. If questions arise as you are reading over the company's literature, call for clarification. Call to make sure you have all available literature. Call about a new product you saw advertised.

Vickie Chepus

a highly skilled colorist who has long managed the technical line of a major manufacturer, has this advice:

"Have your information ready. Confer with your client prior to calling; have a pencil ready. Try to call from a phone where it's quiet, so you can hear. Keep in mind we work in the blind— we don't see, touch, and feel the hair—you are our eyes and hands. We are only as good as the information we get. And remember: If the client changes her mind, you have to call us back! If she wants something else, the same information won't apply . . .

"We are here to help."

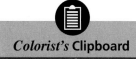

Colorist's Clipboard

Using a manufacturer's toll-free help line

- *Come to the phone prepared, knowing the client's key factors and what you want to achieve, and with swatch chart, paper, and pencil in hand.*

- *Don't ever be afraid to call!*

Client name: *Tipper Moore*

Date: *Today*

Natural base: *6N*

Gray: *5%*

Texture and porosity:

Permed; slightly overporous

Target color:

Bright red-orange, 7 level

Client's comments or ideas:

She loves bright: "My hair couldn't be bright enough."

Colorist's comments or ideas:

Hair is permed. If we don't perm, pre-bleach and tone with the same color.

Pretreatment:

Preshampooed

Formula (regrowth):

Brand name of color, color(s) and volume used

Formula (ends): *Brand and formula*

Application: *Brush application*

Timing: *Minutes on regrowth, ends*

Post-treatment: *Color sealer*

Colorist: *Robin Todd*

Retail: *Shampoo, conditioner, colored shampoo formula*

Result: *Perfect*

If you are ever unsatisfied with a response, give them another chance. Call back and rephrase your question, or request someone else—the Hot Line Supervisor, or the National Education Director. If one of your clients had a problem with your products or services, you would want to know about it. So do manufacturers. The hot line can be a very valuable resource for a salon; use it persistently.

Just one last tip: If you decide not to call the technical line but to ask someone in the salon for an opinion, ask someone who knows more—not less—than you!

CLIENT RECORDS

The importance of keeping good client records really cannot be overstated. There are few things as essential to the smooth operation and growth of a salon than well-kept client records. Good records allow the colorist to plan and execute a program of service for the client, modifying formulas or procedures as needed. This has an inestimable effect on client trust and retention.

Anyone can forget to write something down on occasion, but you are much less likely to forget if you are methodical about your recordkeeping. Use a system, listing the same information in about the same order for every client. Decide what information needs to be noted and establish a format for it, and show everyone in the salon how to do it.

It is a good idea to note the key factors (natural base level, percentage of gray, a porosity factor, and so on), as well as the desired end result.

There may be more than one formula to record (different mixtures for a gray hairline or overporous ends, multiple weave formulas). For corrective clients there will almost always be multiple procedures and formulas. Note the application method and timing in the agreed-upon shorthand ("retouch 25/5," for instance).

And—*so very important*—how satisfactory was the color result? What, if anything, would you do differently next time?

Did you suggest any variations or extra services to the client: a lowlight, a gloss on her length, deeper, lighter, cooler, redder? Your client will remember, but you probably won't, unless you write it down.

Treatments performed and retail products prescribed should also be noted in the client's file. This allows you to evaluate their effect and make any necessary changes.

GETTING THE MOST FROM MANUFACTURERS' SALON CLASSES

A good class is beneficial for so many reasons: learning new things, being reminded of things you used to know and do but forgot, getting answers to nagging questions, voicing pertinent concerns, building esprit de corps and unity, keeping the salon focused, bolstering self-confidence, and creating enthusiasm about services and products!

A poor class, though, makes everyone involved resent the waste of time, and creates negativity: about future programs, about products and services, even about colleagues and the salon itself.

Time is so valuable, and a poor class is such a regrettable loss of time. Simple planning can make all the difference between a good class and a poor class.

Think about what you and your staff need, and ask for it. No one knows the needs of your salon like you do. Tell your sales consultant and the educator what you are looking for—in advance! But, be open to suggestions.

A good educator will have very worthwhile, proven suggestions.

If you have just changed products, always schedule a basic product knowledge class ASAP. Even if your staff is experienced and knowledgeable, always schedule a basic program to ease the transition. You never know what helpful pointers the educator will have! And she will catch on if your staff already knows the basics—she will step up the pace and include more challenging material.

The primary purpose of that first class is to get everyone excited about the change and counteract any apprehension. This is so important. Always make the initial class a simple one—the basics.

No matter what the nature of the color program, allow time for both theory and models. Haircoloring just has to be seen. We hairstylists are very visual people, more moved by pictures than words. If an educator only *talks* about the color product, where is the proof? It is very important to hear the theory first, of course, so designate time for both theory and models. Models should be asked to arrive shortly before the theory portion concludes, out of respect for the models' time, and in order to keep professional information among professionals.

Select appropriate models. Discuss model requirements with the educator well in advance, and follow her suggestions. If it is a basic class, have basic models, not corrective models. The main types of basic color services are: gray coverage, reds, high-lift blonds, highlighting or multishading, and deposit-only haircoloring. Assemble a good mixture of services from those choices, per the educator's instructions.

For a corrective class, the main types of services are: filling (prepigmenting or repigmenting), tint-back, color removal, and contrasting-out unwanted tones. Again, assemble a good mix, per the educator's instructions.

Models should represent the average client. If you ask the most unusual client you have to be a model, what you learn will apply only to that one client. Here I am not talking about fine hair, tenacious or overporous hair, or your standard decolorizing or overlightened highlighting, and so on; these are all within the realm of general experience and are good "teaching models." What I am talking about is the client no one can ever satisfy because she is a chronic attention-seeker, or the physically unwell client whose hair is unpredictable and fragile. A color program should not be totally devoted to one highly individualistic color problem. That's a waste of time. A better way of getting help with such a client is to discuss it with the educator and try to arrange for him or her to be present at the client's next appointment. This way the educator has a fair chance to deal with the atypical nature of the client, and you are not wasting the time of everyone in the salon.

Select the appropriate number of models. Follow the educator's instructions on this point. Too many models can make a class chaotic or repetitive. Too few can leave you wondering what you learned. For a typical four-hour class, three models is often ideal.

The salon staff should be actively involved in the analysis, formulation, mixing, application, rinsing, and review of models. A good educator will guide the staff in analysis and formulation, then assist in mixing, application, and rinsing, but will have your staff do most of the work. This will make the class more meaningful, more interesting, and more confidence-inspiring for

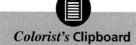

Colorist's Clipboard

Information to be included on the client record

• Key factors (base level, percentage of gray, any porosity factor, and so on).

• Desired result.

• Formula, application, timing.

• Your satisfaction with the result.

• Any changes or additional services you recommended.

• Any clues she gave you about what she likes or dislikes, what she might want in the future, and so on.

• Treatment services; at-home maintenance.

your stylists. Be sure every stylist sees every model before any color is applied, and do not allow models to leave until everyone has seen the results. If color is applied before all the stylists get a chance to look at the hair, or if the model leaves without a proper review, then the salon has not learned from that application; it was essentially a waste of time and product.

Always confirm a few days prior with the educator and models. The educator should take the initiative to confirm the class with you, but if not, call. Remind your models, too, and make sure they know how long they can expect to be in the salon. A simple phone call can save a lot of aggravation.

Give the educator your undivided attention. If you are going to have a class, then *have a class.* Do not accept clients during class time, do not spend undue time on the phone, do not conduct business with salespeople. And have your entire staff present. If you are going to take your time and the time of your staff to have a class, then make it count. Take it seriously and treat it as valuable.

Share education with other salons. Invite other salons to come to your class. Both the educator and your fellow salons will appreciate this. It makes for a more stimulating class, and it will help bridge the competition gap! Joint participation puts you on friendlier terms with local salons, and that's good for everyone's business.

Ask distributor or manufacturer reps to tell you about programs in local salons that you may attend. If you or someone in the salon has a special interest in certain products, needs additional information, or is just very highly motivated, this is a way of getting extra education without involving the entire staff.

Colorist's Clipboard

Getting the most from salon color classes

- *Tell the educator in advance what you need from the class; listen to his or her suggestions.*

- *Allow time for both theory and models and select appropriate models.*

- *Confirm the class a few days prior with both educator and models.*

- *Don't let the educator do all the work! Learn by doing.*

- *Look at all models carefully before any color goes on, and review the results afterwards. That is how you train your eye.*

- *Give the educator your undivided attention.*

- *Share education with other salons.*

RECOMMENDED BOOKS, VIDEOS, PROFESSIONAL ORGANIZATIONS, AND EVENTS

On the subject of color in general—not haircoloring, but color generally—there is an abundance of information and just a few key works are listed below. There are relatively few books, however, on the subjects of hair structure and haircoloring. If you are searching for an answer to a specific question about haircoloring, periodicals may be of assistance, especially *Journal of the Society of Cosmetic Chemists, International Journal of Cosmetic Science,* and *Cosmetics & Toiletries.*

The titles listed here may be available at your local public library, either on the shelf or through interlibrary loan. Color theory books are most likely to be found in large public libraries or in the libraries of colleges that have fine arts curricula. Scientific references are most likely to be found in college science or medical libraries. Call or visit the libraries of nearby campuses, or contact a bookstore or the publisher.

There aren't many generic haircoloring videos, but a few are listed here. Contact the maker of the video to obtain more information or a copy.

On the Subject of Color:

Birren, F. *Color and Human Response.* New York, NY: Van Nostrand Reinhold, 1978. Color theories and theorists, the nature of light, and the optics and psychology of color.

Birren, F. *Principles of Color.* West Chester, PA: Schiffer, 1987. A superb overview of color theory.

Chevreul, M.E. *The Principles of Harmony and Contrast of Colors.* Edited by F. Birren. New York, NY: Van Nostrand Reinhold,

1967. Theories of the great nineteenth-century French color authority, Michel Eugene Chevreul. This edition is enhanced by Birren's helpful commentary.

Cole, A. *Color.* New York, NY: Dorling Kindersley, 1993. Introduction to the painter's use of color. Appealing simplicity; visual appeal.

Itten, J. *The Art of Color.* Edited by F. Birren. New York, NY: Van Nostrand Reinhold, 1970. Theories of Johannes Itten, 1888–1967, Bauhaus master, one of the great color teachers of the modern age.

Munsell, A.H. *A Color Notation.* Rev. ed. Baltimore, MD: Munsell Color Co., 1946. American painter and theorist Albert Munsell, 1858–1918. The Munsell system of color notation is the basis for our level system classification of haircoloring.

Parramon, J.M. *The Book of Color.* New York, NY: Watson-Guptill, 1993. Contemporary painter and teacher Jose Parramon presents the history, theory, and use of color in this beautifully illustrated work.

On the Science of Hair and Haircoloring Products:

Balsam, M.S. and E. Sagarin, eds. *Cosmetics: Science and Technology.* 2nd ed. New York, NY: Wiley Interscience, 1972. The history of haircoloring and bleaches is woven through the article by Florence E. Wall (pages 279–343).

Robbins, C.R. *Chemical and Physical Behavior of Human Hair.* New York, NY: Springer-Verlag, 1988. There is some difficult reading in this book, but it is very worthwhile.

Schoon, D.D. *Hair Structure and Chemistry Simplified.* Rev. ed. Albany, NY: Milady Publishing, 1993. Biology and chemistry written for cosmetologists.

Spencer, P. *Hair Coloring, A Hands-On Approach.* Albany, NY: Milady Publishing, 1990. Written by a cosmetology instructor; emphasis on color experiments and chemistry; richly detailed.

Zviak, C., ed. *The Science of Hair Care.* New York: Marcel Dekker, 1986. Exceptionally informative. Written for a broader audience than most of the scientific references, which are usually intended strictly for chemists or strictly for cosmetologists.

For Teachers:

Nizetich, A. *Teaching Hair Coloring, A Step-by-Step Guide to Building Props.* Albany, NY: Milady Publishing, 1993. Of interest to anyone who teaches (instructors, educators, color directors). Imaginative; lots of how-to photos.

Videos:

The Primary Series. Scott Cole and Linda Yodice, of Colorcutting USA, Carefree, Arizona, pair five basic cuts and foil techniques. Cole is a former Sassoon Artistic Director; he and Yodice are well-known educators.

PUREducation Haircoloring Methods. Salon Visage, Knoxville, Tennessee. Volumes I, II and III are basic and creative foil techniques by respected educator Belinda Gambuzza.

Double Your Haircolor Income. Mark D. Foley Enterprises Limited, Calgary, Alberta, Canada. Marketing advice specifically pertaining to haircoloring services. Foley is a salon owner and marketing strategist.

Color Smart. Bobby J's Inc., Pittsburgh, Pennsylvania. Video and manual cover the basics of color, color correction, and special effects coloring.

Robin Todd

head of the color department at Ann Bray's The Masters Salon, Huntsville, Alabama:

"Of course we'll write down the natural base and do the consultation. I like to write down certain things they say, like 'I hate red,' 'I turn brassy,' 'Those beiges look red to me,' so that I can bring it up later. They are always so thrilled I remembered (and I don't remember at all; we do too many clients to remember). I also write down any ideas I have for them—if I see them in a gold tone, whatever—then when I have their trust I can suggest it . . .

"We write down anything we think is important. Whether we preshampooed, mixed a colored shampoo . . . the order that the weave formulas were applied . . . what was done and who did it, and the date."

Professional Events and Organizations:

International Haircolor Exchange, 1-800-COLOR-55. Nonprofit organization run by colorists. IHE "event" is limited to 500 attendees and held in a different city each year; showcases generic color techniques by independent artists and new technology by manufacturers (no product knowledge). Newsletter every other month. Founded 1986.

Haircolor USA, 1-800-331-5706. Large yearly color show. Education by both independent artists and manufacturers, including product knowledge classes. Traditionally held in Miami, Florida, in June. Founded 1987.

National Cosmetology Association, 1-800-527-1683. The oldest (founded 1921) and largest (32,000 members) organization of licensed cosmetologists in the United States.

NCA goals are education and legislation. Twice-yearly trend releases; 500 affiliates meet locally.

Colour Connection, 1-905-569-1065. The first Canadian haircolorists' group. Yearly show with both manufacturer and independent education. Quarterly newsletter. Founded 1993.

Intercoiffure, 1-412-342-6090 or 1-504-288-9003. Prestigious international group. Unlike other organizations, events are by invitation only and prospective members must qualify for membership via a screening process. Members share business and artistic know-how. Founded in Paris, 1912; came to the United States in 1933.

American Board of Certified Master Haircolorists (AB of CMH), 1-310-547-0814. Nonprofit organization, founded 1995 to establish a higher standard for haircolorists.

appendices

A

coloring chemically relaxed hair

African-American hair, Caucasian hair, Native-American, Japanese, Hispanic—haircoloring doesn't know the difference. Hair is all basically the same structurally. "Hair is hair," Reginald Mitchell says. Hair that has been treated with a sodium hydroxide relaxer, though, has been significantly altered (structurally changed) and requires more care, much like permanently waved hair needs more care. This is an excerpt of a conversation with Reginald, Director of Training for a major manufacturer specializing in products for African-American hair.

Q. Do you have any specific recommendations for coloring African-American hair?

A. African-American hair is usually much dryer than the hair of the Caucasian client. However, with any chemical the hair should be in a relatively healthy state before a chemical application of any type.

Q. How many levels of lift do you advise for relaxed hair?

A. On chemically treated hair, the first factor is the condition of the hair. The second factor is the natural color of the hair.

Q. Would you lift relaxed hair four levels?

A. If it is in good condition, yes! Just as permed hair runs the gamut from healthy to abused, so does

relaxed hair. Most of the time, perms and relaxers create additional porosity but do not excessively damage hair, and most clients wearing sodium hydroxide relaxers can be colored with permanent haircoloring. If the hair isn't in good condition, though, deposit-only products are gentler. Semi-permanent haircoloring, which does not use hydrogen peroxide, or no-lift demi-permanents, which use very low-volume developers, are especially gentle choices because it is the lifting process that is most damaging to hair. Mistreated, brittle, breakable hair should not be colored at all, of course; it should be conditioned.

Bobby J. Hunt, owner of Bobby J's in Pittsburgh, Pennsylvania (4 salons, 70 employees) says, "I look at relaxed hair as presoftened hair. It will process quicker. The cuticle is already standing up.

"I find we can move the hair up four levels without damaging it, if the hair has been properly treated . . . At the end of your color process did you take all the precautions? Did you eliminate all residue, did you condition it properly, is she using the proper maintenance products? If I am orienting my customers to what it takes to maintain a healthy head of hair with color, they have no problem at all. And we've been doing this for years. The key is to use a color that is less damaging. You have to feel around as a designer and find the color that will work best for you. Any color will work, but will it leave the hair in good condition? Shop around for the right product."

Charles Gregory, who owns a salon in Atlanta, Georgia, talks about the importance of considering how relaxer clients maintain their hair, before deciding which color process is best for them. "If they have a relaxer and they curl their hair more than twice a week, I usually won't recommend permanent color," he says. "I find out what kind of activities they're into. If they're athletic or they work out, and they're shampooing more than twice a week and using hot rollers or curling irons every other day, that takes a lot of moisture and elasticity out of relaxed hair. I don't really recommend they get permanent color but I will do semi-permanent."

a brief history of haircoloring

A BRIEF HISTORY OF HAIRCOLORING

Haircoloring is known to have been practiced at least 4600 years, which is almost as far back as historical records go. The culture credited with first coloring hair is ancient Egypt, where the use of henna dates from about 2600 B.C. Oxidation coloring as we know it has its origins in the late nineteenth century, when hydrogen peroxide and synthetic dyes came into use. Single-process coloring came into use around 1950.

Vegetable Dyes

Botanicals represent the oldest and most diverse source of haircoloring. Henna, an ornamental shrub native to India, Egypt, and the Middle and Far East, was the first substance used to color hair. Like many vegetable dyes, it has been used ever since. The leaves of henna, which contain a strong red-orange colorant, are dried, crushed, and mixed with hot water to make a dye paste.

Other age-old plant dyes include the yellow of chamomile flowers, the blue-green of the indigo plant, and wood extracts—walnut shells, for example, with which a brown dye bath is made. The gallnuts of white oak were used by the ancient Chinese to make dye packs. Many other plant dyes have served as haircolorants: extracts of logwood, madder root, saffron, elderberry, rhubarb, radish, willow, and sage, among others. The Cheyenne word for the wild begonia of the American west is *ma'i tuk ohe'*, or "red maker"; it was used to redden hair as well as quills and feathers.[1]

An herbalist's book dated 1636 says this of sumac: "The decoction of the leaves maketh haires blacke."[2] The Ladies Dictionary, 1694, provides this advice: "a mixture of bark of oak root, green husks of walnuts, the deepest and oldest red wine and oil of myrtle will turn any coloured hair as black as jet."[3]

Metallic Dyes

Metals commonly used as dye materials include lead, silver, and copper. It may have been the ancient Greeks who created the original progressive metallic tint, at least 2000 years ago. The ancient Greeks and Romans darkened their tresses with lead combs dipped in wine vinegar, which made essentially the same lead acetate found in today's metallic tint. Traces of lead clung to the hair as it was passed through the acidified comb, "restoring" color to what had been gray. Lead combs were used in Europe centuries later for the same purpose.

The first-century folk-historian Pliny the Elder notes a number of methods of haircoloring used by his Roman countrymen. Most famous are these directions for metallic tint: "If one be disposed to colour the hair of the head black, let him . . . put as many horse-leeches as a sextar [approximately one pint] will hold, in two sextars of vinegar, and let them putrify in a vessel of lead [for sixty days]; and when they be reduced into the form of a liniment, to annoint the hair in the sunshine."[4] Pliny adds that this dye is so potent, the subject's teeth might also turn black unless he or she keeps a cheekful of oil in his or her mouth for the duration of the "annointing"!

1 Kindscher, K. Medicinal Wild Plants of the Prairie (Lawrence, KS: University Press of Kansas, 1992), p. 278.

2 Ibid., p 186.
3 De Courtais, G., Women's Headdress and Hairstyles (B.T. Batsford, 1986), p. 70.
4 Pliny, Natural History. P. Holland, trans., J.M. Cohen, ed. (Carbondate, Il: Southern Illinois University Press, 1962), p. 346.

Natural Lighteners

The women of ancient Rome practiced, and probably discovered, bleaching. Envious of the blond-haired Gauls that Caesar enslaved, they learned to lighten their hair with wood ash mixed with vinegar, or ash and goat tallow, which is lye soap—first invented for the purpose of blonding, not bathing. The ancient Greeks, both male and female, also lightened their hair with wood ash, then used a vegetable rinse (a sort of tea derived from flowers) and sunlight to blond it further.

Variations on these methods of bleaching persisted until the advent of chemistry in the 1800s. Many Renaissance and Post-Renaissance cultures used wood ash, for its high-alkalinity and potassium content, to lighten hair. The sixteenth-century artist Titian portrayed the women of Venice as red-blonds ("Titian blonds") because they soaked their hair with a kind of potassium lye, then sat in the sun with their hair draped over the broad rims of open-topped hats. (Such methods were harsh and of relatively limited effect.)

Powders

The lavish, powdered hair of the seventeenth and eighteenth centuries—à la Marie Antoinette—was an early form of temporary haircoloring. It seems curious today, but the application of powders to hair (and wigs) made sticky with animal fat was common in Europe for hundreds of years. This practice originated in ancient times with the use of powdered gold (an extravagance revived by Napoleon's court in the 1850s, to use up the surplus created by the American gold rush), but the powders usually consisted of much humbler fare, such as wheat starch, potato starch, or chalk, over a pomade of lard.

Chemical Lighteners and Oxidation Dyes

The advent of chemistry as a scientific study, in the late 1700s, opened up a new age for haircoloring. Chemistry has brought about most of today's lighteners and dyes:

1818—the discovery of hydrogen peroxide (H_2O_2)

Mid-1800s—discovery of the first synthetic-organic (coal-tar) dyes (pyrogallol, 1845; mauvine, 1856

1854—the invention of the first amino dye, metaphenylenediamine

1863—the invention of paraphenylenediamine (PPD)

1867—hydrogen peroxide used in hair-bleaching demonstrations at the Paris Exposition by French hairdresser, Leon Hugo, and an English chemist, E. H. Thiellay

Mid-1880s—French patent issued for the use of PPD in haircoloring; German patents issued for the use of aminophenols and nitroderivatives in haircoloring

Mid-1890s—a variety of amino haircoloring products in use in Europe and America

Noteworthy amino colors of the early 1900s included Gaston Boudou's Inecto (Boudou was a hairdresser with salons in London and Paris) and Eugene Schueller's Aureole. Schueller, a French chemist, founded L'Oréal). These products represented a big improvement over what had been previously available, but permanent haircoloring still had a long way to go.

Oxidation color was all double-process until the middle of the twentieth century. Tints were not capable of lightening; the hair was prepared for tinting by a preliminary bleaching to presoften or lighten it. (The hairstylist used a bleaching solution first, shampooed, then applied the dye solution.)

Another of the first single-process colors was Miss Clairol, introduced at the New York IBS in February of 1950. The book *50 Colorful Years* (Stein, M., Clairol, 1982, p.15) describes the launch:

"For four days, standing-room-only audiences of hairdressers and salon owners watched spellbound as the Clairol staff performed complete color treatments in 20 minutes. To assure the audience that no tricks were taking place behind the scenes, technicians performed the entire coloring process on stage—using buckets of water to rinse the models' hair." (Single-process color was so revolutionary that hairdressers were reluctant to believe it was possible! Two of the people responsible for Miss Clairol were hairdresser Vern Silberman—Miss Vern—and the late biochemist, Dr. Bernard Lustig.)

Single-process color as we know it today has only been in use since about 1950. Early versions of several of today's leading single-process, permanent color products, including Wella's *Kolestone*, Clairol's *Miss Clairol*, and *Lapinal* (now owned by Redken), were introduced in 1950 or shortly thereafter.

appendix c

haircoloring and cancer myths

HAIRCOLORING AND CANCER MYTHS

The question of whether hair dyes contribute to the incidence of various cancers has been copiously studied, with sometimes mixed results. The most recent and best studies, however, show no relationship between hair dyes and cancer.

Over the years, certain dye components have been eliminated from products because of suspected carcinogenicity. Harvard Medical School's Chief of Preventive Medicine, Dr. Charles Hennekens, says hair dyes were unfairly vilified by early studies that involved application of "humongous" quantities of dyes to animals and did not account for cigarette use among human subjects. In 1985, Dr. R. Wilson of Harvard wrote that the risk posed by the worst discontinued dye was the equivalent of smoking a total of six cigarettes over a lifetime.

Two of the most recent and most comprehensive studies cleared hair dyes of any association with cancer. A study completed in 1993 showed no link between hair dyes and cancers of the mouth, breast, lung, bladder, or cervix. In 1994, the largest, longest-running study ever conducted concluded that neither was there any link between hair dyes and Hodgkin's lymphoma, non-Hodgkin's lymphoma, multiple myeloma, or leukemias.

Information on these and other studies is readily available from the American Cancer Society (1-800-227-2345), or the Cancer Information Service of the National Cancer Institute (1-800-422-6237).

a few final words

Haircoloring is really a pretty simple equation: the key factors, plus the formula, equals the end result.

Key Factors + Formula = Result.

To get the desired end result, then, you must be familiar with two things: the hair you are coloring, and the haircoloring product you are using. You must do a good analysis, and your product knowledge must be up to snuff.

Natural base level is foremost among the key factors. If there is little or no gray, average texture, normal porosity and no existing tint, then all that matters is the natural base level. As often as not, however, there will be other factors to consider.

We say that natural pigment is 50 percent of the color result. (The formula is the other 50 percent.) In reality, that statement is an oversimplification, but it does convey the importance of knowing about natural pigment: identification of natural base level, percentage of gray, and dominant underlying color.

As far as the formula is concerned, it has two facets: lift (the developer, mostly) and deposit (the dyes, mostly). So, to write good formulas, you must understand developer selection, and you must be familiar with color theory and with the pigments in those tubes or bottles on the dispensary shelves.

WHAT EVERY COLOR CLIENT WANTS

It doesn't matter if it is virgin color, retouch, a conversion, a correction, creative haircoloring, demi-permanent, permanent, or double-process, every color service has the same basic goals.

Every color client wants:

1. **the right color**
2. **which lasts as long as it is supposed to, and**
3. **which leaves her hair in good condition.**

To the client, the right haircolor is the one she told you she wanted—the one she understood you would give her. From a technical perspective, the right color is the desired level and tone, from scalp to ends and front to back. Good color can only be achieved through proper analysis, communication, formulation, and application.

Haircoloring should last as long as it is supposed to last. If you tell your client it will largely fade away before her next cut, it should. If you tell her it will hold true until her retouch, it should. If it doesn't, then the formula or procedure should be adjusted accordingly (or you should adjust your client's expectations).

All haircoloring renders the hair somewhat more porous. A good colorist keeps the damage to a minimum by choosing the gentlest means of achieving the desired end result, performing any necessary treatments and prescribing proper retail. The better the condition of the client's hair, the better the color will look and hold—the more numerous the client's cut, color, and perm options—and the easier the haircolorist's job.

THE ART OF HAIRCOLORING

Haircoloring cannot be reduced entirely to a science. There are many things about coloring hair that are given to objective analysis and systemization, as this and other books demonstrate, but some aspects of haircoloring defy any exact system, and sometimes even exact expression. Dwight Miller, creator of a well-known haircutting system, says, "Systems are good, because then you know what you know; the problem is, you don't know what you don't know." The system doesn't necessarily capture it all, in other words.

Professional haircoloring is an art as well as a science, from artful communication to artful application. Haircoloring done really well is a creative process that may not be entirely preplanned or done in a conventional way. Done really well, it is done by the rules, but also by feel, and a feel for color is gained only through experience. Technical proficiency is really the beginning—not the totality—of expertise; there are many techniques to master, and more to invent.

Faber Birren, in an introduction to one of his books, said: "This book seeks to inspire, not conformance to color law (where it may happen to exist), but to knowledgeable release for the artist and designer."[1] Johannes Itten called certain laws of color "inexorable," and said, "We can be released from subjective bondage only through knowledge and awareness of objective principles."[2]

This book was written to promote knowledge of objective principles, as well as the curiosity and creativity that knowledge inspires.

---

1 Birren, F., Principles of Color (West Chester, PA: Schiffer, 1987), p. 5.
2 Itten, J., The Elements of Color (New York, NY: Van Nostrand Reinhold, 1970), pp. 94, 97.

references

American Cancer Society Cancer Response System, publication number 2284.

Birren, F. *Color and Human Response.* New York, NY: Van Nostrand Reinhold, 1978.

Birren, F. *Color Perception in Art.* West Chester, PA: Schiffer, 1986.

Birren, F. *Principles of Color.* West Chester, PA: Schiffer, 1987.

Bradfield, R.B. Effect of undernutrition upon hair growth, in *Hair Research.* Edited by C.E. Orfanos, W. Montagna and G. Stuttgen. New York, NY: Springer-Verlag, 1981. 251–256.

Branley, F. *Color, From Rainbows to Lasers.* New York, NY: Thomas Y. Crowell, 1978.

Bublin, J.G. and D.F. Thompson. 1992. Drug-induced haircolour changes, *Journal of Clinical Pharmacy and Therapeutics* 17:297–302.

Burnett, J. 1989. Copper. *Cutis* 43(4):322.

Burnie, D. *Light.* New York, NY: Dorling Kindersley, 1992.

Calnan, C. Adverse reactions to hair products, in *The Science of Hair Care.* Edited by C. Zviak. New York, NY: Marcel Dekker, 1986. 409–412.

Cannell, D.W. *Hair Around the World.* New York, NY: Redken Laboratories.

Chevreul, M.E. *The Principles of Harmony and Contrast of Colors.* Edited by F. Birren. New York, NY: Van Nostrand Reinhold, 1967.

Cline, D.J. 1988. Changes in haircolor, *Dermatalogic Clinics* 6(2):295–303.

Cole, A. *Color.* New York, NY: Dorling Kindersley, 1993.

Comaish, J.S. Hair growth in disorders of metabolism, in *Hair Research.*

267-273. Edited by C.E. Orfanos, W. Montagna and G. Stuttgen. New York, NY: Springer-Verlag, 1981. 267–273.

Cone, E. et al. 1991. Testing human hair for drugs of abuse. II. Identification of unique cocaine metabolites in hair of drug abusers and evaluation of decontamination procedures, *Journal of Analytical Toxicology* 15:250–255.

Contini, M. *Fashion from Ancient Egypt to the Present Day.* New York, NY: Odyssey Press, 1965.

Corbett, J. 1984. Chemistry of hair colorant processes—Science as an aid to formulation and development, *Journal of the Society of Cosmetic Chemists* 35:297–310.

Corbett, J. 1991. Haircoloring processes, *Cosmetics & Toiletries* 106:53–57.

Draelos, Z. 1991. Hair cosmetics, *Dermatologic Clinics* 9:19–27.

Evans, R. *An Introduction to Color.* New York, NY: John Wiley and Sons, 1959.

Fair, N. and B.S. Gupta. 1982. Effects of chlorine on friction and morphology of human hair, *Journal of the Society of Cosmetic Chemists* 33:229–242.

Fair N.B. and B.S. Gupta. 1988. The chlorine hair interaction. III. Effect of combining chlorination with cosmetic treatments on hair properties, *Journal of the Society of Cosmetic Chemists* 39:93–105.

Feinland, R. and W. Vaniotis. 1986. Clinical evaluation of haircolor, *Cosmetics and Tolietries* 101:63–66.

Fisher, A. 1989. Management of hairdressers sensitized to hair dyes or permanent wave solutions, *Cutis* 43:316–318.

Fisher, A. and A. Dooms-Goossens. 1976. Persulfate hair bleach reactions, *Archives of Dermatology* 112: 1407–1409.

Gerrard, W.A. 1989. The measurement of haircolour, *International Journal of Cosmetic Science* 11:97–101.

Gerstner, K. *The Forms of Color*. Cambridge, MA: MIT Press, 1986.

Grodstein, F., et al. 1994. A prospective study of permanent hair dye use and hematopoietic cancer, *Journal of the National Cancer Institute* 86:1466–1470.

Guerra, L., et al. 1992. Contact dermatitis in hairdresser's clients, *Contact Dermatitis* 26:108–111.

Hammershoy, O. 1980. Standard patch test results in 3,225 consecutive Danish patients from 1973 to 1977, *Contact Dermatitis* 6:263–268.

Hardy, A. *Colorimetry*. Cambridge, MA: MIT Press, 1936.

Hope, A. and M. Walch. *The Color Compendium*. New York, NY: Van Nostrand Reinhold, 1990.

Itten, J. *The Art of Color*. Edited by F. Birren. New York, NY: Van Nostrand Reinhold, 1970.

Jachowicz, J. 1987. Hair damage and attempts to its repair, *Journal of the Society of Cosmetic Chemists* 38:263–286.

Kelly, S. and V.N.E. Robinson. 1982. The effect of grooming on the hair cuticle, *Journal of the Society of Cosmetic Chemists* 33:203–215.

Kindsher, K. Medicinal *Wild Plants of the Prairie*. Lawrence, KS: University Press of Kansas, 1992.

Korman, L. *Beauty by the decades* 1878–1907. American Salon August 1997, 110–113.

Mahnke, F. and R. Mahnke. *Color and Light in Man-made Environments*. New York, NY: Van Nostrand Reinhold, 1987.

McKenzie, J. 1978. Alteration of the zinc and copper concentration of hair, *American Journal of Clinical Nutrition* 31:470–476.

Munsell, A.H. *A Color Notation*. Rev. ed. Baltimore, MD: Munsell Color Co., 1946.

Nassau, K. *The Physics and Chemistry of Color*. New York, NY: Wiley-Interscience, 1983.

Newton, I. *Optics*. Repr. in *Great Books*. Chicago, IL: Encyclopaedia Brittanica, 1952.

O'Donoghue, M.N. Hair cosmetics, *Dermatologic Clinics* 5:619–626.

Ortonne, J.P. and G. Prota. 1993. Hair melanins and haircolor: Ultrastructural and biochemical aspects, *Journal of Investigative Dermatology* 101:82S–89S12.

Ortonne, J.P. and J. Thivolet. Hair melanin and haircolor, in *Hair Research*. Edited by C.E. Orfanos, W. Montagna, and G. Stuttgen. New York, NY: Springer-Verlag, 1981. 146–162.

Pande, C. and J. Jachowicz. 1993. Hair photodamage—Measurement and prevention, *Journal of the Society of Cosmetic Chemists* 44:109–122.

Parramon, J.M. *The Book of Color*. New York, NY: Watson-Guptill, 1993.

Pliny. *Natural History*. Translation by P. Holland. Edited by J.M. Cohen. Carbondale, IL: Southern Illinois University Press, 1962.

Pohl, S. 1988. Chemistry of hair dyes, *Cosmetics & Toiletries*. 103:57–66.

Powitt, A.H. *Hair Structure and Chemistry Simplified.* Albany, NY: Milady Publishing, 1977.

Prota, G. *Melanins and Melanogenesis.* New York, NY: Academic Press, 1992.

Rainwater, C. *Light and Color.* New York, NY: Golden Press, 1971.

Rattee, I.D. 1978. Color in cosmetics, in *Cosmetic Science.* Edited by M. Breuer. London, UK: Academic Press. 189–200.

Robbins, C. *Chemical and Physical Behavior of Human Hai.,* New York, NY: Springer-Verlag, 1988.

Robins, A.H. *Biological Perspectives on Human Pigmentation.* Cambridge, UK: Cambridge University Press, 1991. 89–91.

Rovner, S. "Hair dye not linked to cancer development," *Washington Post,* final ed., 11 October 1994, Z5.

Schoon, D.D. *Hair Structure and Chemistry Simplified,* rev. ed. Albany, NY: Milady Publishing, 1993.

Solomon, E., et al. *Human Anatomy and Physiology,* 2nd ed. Philadelphia, PA: Saunders College Publishing, 1990.

Spencer, P. *Hair Coloring, A Hands-On Approach.* Albany, NY: Milady Publishing, 1990.

Stein, M. *50 Colorful Years.* New York, NY: Clairol, 1982. Courtesy of Leland Hirsch.

Trasko, M. *Daring Do's.* New York, NY: Flammarion, 1994.

Tsujino Y., et al. 1991. Haircoloring and waving using oxidases, *Journal of the Society of Cosmetic Chemists* 42:273–282.

Valkovic, V. and D. Rendic. Studies on trace elements in human hair by x-ray emission spectroscopy, in *Hair Research.* Edited by C.E. Orfanos, W. Montagna, and G. Stuttgen. New York, NY: Springer-Verlag, 1981. 129–132.

Van Scott, E.J. Drug induced alopecia, in *Hair Research.* Edited by C.E. Orfanos, W. Montagna, and G. Stuttgen. New York, NY: Springer-Verlag, 1981. 469–474.

Wall, F.E. Bleaches, haircolorings and dye removers, in *Cosmetics: Science and Technology.* Edited by M.S. Balsam and E. Sagarin. New York, NY: Wiley Interscience, 1972. 279–343.

Watt, N.B. *Text Book of the Del-Mar School of Beauty Culture.* Detroit, MI: 1932. Courtesy of David Pressley.

Wilson, R. Risks posed by various components of hair dyes, *Archives of Dermatological Research* 278:165–170.

Wolfram, L.J. The reactivity of human hair, a review, in *Hair Research.* Edited by C.E. Orfanos, W. Montagna, and G. Stuttgen. New York, NY: Springer-Verlag, 1981. 479–500.

Wolfram, L.J. and L. Albrecht. 1987. Chemical- and photo-bleaching of brown and red hair. *Journal of the Society of Cosmetic Chemists* 82:179–191.

Wolfram, L.J., K. Hall, and I. Hui. 1970. The mechanism of hair bleaching, *Journal of the Society of Cosmetic Chemists* 21:875–900.

Wolfram, L.J. and M. Lindeman. 1971. Some observations on the hair cuticle, *Journal of the Society of Cosmetic Chemists* 22:839–850.

Zahn, H. S. Hilterhaus, and A. Strubmann. Bleaching and permanent waving aspects of hair research, *Journal of the Society of Cosmetic Chemists* 37:159–175.

Zviak, C. Hair bleaching; Haircoloring: non-oxidation coloring; and Oxidation coloring, in *The Science of Hair Care.* New York, NY: Marcel Dekker, 1986. 213–286.

Zviak, C. and R.P.R. Dawber. Hair structure, function and physicochemical properties, in *The Science of Hair Care.* New York, NY: Marcel Dekker, 1986. 1–48.

glossary/index

Abused rejection: the selective rejection of artificial pigment due to damaged, overporous condition. Hair that is overporous tends to reject warm artificial pigment and absorb ash artificial pigment. Formulas for extremely overporous hair are therefore warmer (more gold, more red, less ash, or void of ash). See *porosity, overporous hair, extreme overporosity,* and *moderate overporosity.*   **p. 27**

Acid rinse: an instant conditioner with a mild acid pH, used after haircoloring services to neutralize any remaining alkalinity. (Bleaches and haircoloring are alkaline in pH.)   **p. 83**

Alkali: a substance having a pH of greater than 7.   **p. 38**

Alkaline: having a pH of greater than 7.   **p. 35**

Allergen: a substance that causes an allergic reaction.   **p. 76**

Allergenic: tending to induce allergy. A substance that causes allergic reactions more commonly than do other substances is said to be allergenic. *Allergenicity* is the allergenic quality of a substance.   **p. 76**

Allergy: adverse physiological reaction (such as hives or rash) to a specific substance.   **p. 76**

Amino acids: the "building blocks," or main components, of proteins. Amino acids are the main components of keratin.   **p. 16**

Ammonia: an alkaline compound used in haircoloring as a catalyst to oxidation and/or to give the haircoloring an alkaline pH (which swells the hairshaft and increases penetration). Ammonia is a compound of nitrogen and hydrogen (NH_3).   **p. 37**

Aniline-derivative haircoloring: haircoloring having dyes synthetically derived from coal tar. Oxidation haircoloring contains aniline derivative dyes, also called *amino dyes* and *synthetic organic dyes.*   **p. 37**

Balancing: see *browning-out.*

Bleach-and-tone: a two-process color service in which the hair is first lightened with scalp bleach (called the *bleach-out*), then colored (*toning*). Toners may be labelled as such, or can be any low- or no-peroxide haircoloring, formulated appropriately for prelightened hair.   **p. 23**

Bleach-out: a color service in which natural haircolor is bleached to a light stage, usually followed by toning; to lighten with scalp bleach.   **p. 96**

Blend: to merge different colors in the hair, or to create a harmonious mix of colors. Here are two examples: 1) using semi- or demi-permanent color on previously highlighted hair, to blend the colored and uncolored portions; 2) using semi- or demi-permanent color to blend gray, which will cover some of the gray, tone some, and leave some still visible.   **p. 91**

Booster: broadly, anything added-in to increase lightening capability. Usually refers to the powder packet added to scalp bleach (oil bleach) to increase lightening, which is also called an *activator* or *protinator.* Cream boosters may be provided for use with permanent haircoloring, as well.   **p. 96**

Browning-out: to mute or neutralize an unwanted tone with its complement or with a neutral color. Sometimes also called *balancing* or *overtoning.*   **p. 11**

Carcinogenicity: the cancer-causing quality of a substance (*carcinogenic* means cancer-causing).   **p. 168**

Catalyst: a substance that speeds up a chemical reaction or increases the effect of other substances.   **p. 37**

Chelating shampoo: a shampoo containing chelating agents, used to remove unwanted minerals from hair.   **p. 123**

Chelators, chelating agents: substances in shampoos and treatments that react with (combine with) metals (minerals), to draw out minerals from the hair. Common chelators are EDTA (ethylene diamine tetracetic acid) and DTPA (diethelene triamine pentaacetic acid).
p. 123

Chlorine green: see *copper green.*

Clarifying products: shampoos or treatments designed to remove foreign substances, especially cosmetic build-ups, from hair; also called *detoxifying* products.   **p. 125**

Coarse hair: hair that is coarser than average (the individual hairs are of greater than average diameter). Coarse hair tends to take longer to penetrate and color than hair of average texture. Coarse hair has more cortical area (and therefore more melanin) than average hair. See *texture.*   **p. 24**

Cold shaft: the midshaft; the portion of the strand away from the heat of the scalp.   **p. 28**

Color: a physical, chemical, optical, and psychological phenomenon; our eyes interpret reflected light as color. The color of an object depends upon its pigmentation and surface qualities, what light is available, and the vision of whomever is looking at it.   **p. 4**

Color album: an assortment of photos or magazine pictures of artificially colored hair, including solid colors, highlighting, special effects, before-and-afters, and so on, arranged in book or album form and used during color consultations to aid client communication.   **p. 54**

Color analysis: a service to determine which colors of clothing, make-up, and haircoloring best complement natural coloring, usually done by draping the client with fabric of different colors. There are numerous methods of color analysis, some simple, some complex.   **p. 55**

Color-and-shine products: pigmented glosses that contain direct dyes (no developer required) and have a "conditioning" effect (shining and bulking up the hair); may be processed with or without heat, and may last temporarily or indefinitely.   **p. 34**

Color filler: a haircoloring product or formula used to prepigment previously lightened or overporous hair, replacing missing underlying pigment, compensating for overporosity, and preparing the hair for even acceptance of whatever haircoloring follows.   **p. 23**

Color processing machines: infrared lights, steamers, and ozone machines, used to accelerate haircoloring processes.   **p. 83**

Color removal: partial or complete removal of artificial haircoloring.   **p. 119**

Color removers: products designed to remove artificial haircoloring, also called *decolorizing products.* Color removers intended for use with oxidation haircoloring are usually mild bleaches which are also capable of lightening natural pigment. Color removers intended for use with semi-permanent haircoloring are usually oil and/or isopropyl alcohol based solvents.   **p. 119**

Color shaker: a plastic bowl with a lid, for mixing haircoloring by shaking rather than stirring.   **p. 78**

Color spectrum: the band of colors seen when white light is separated by wavelength.

Rainbows display the color spectrum, as does light passing through a prism. The spectral colors are red, orange, yellow, green, blue, and violet, each representing different wavelengths of light.   **p. 4**

Color wheel: a circle that shows graphically how hues relate to each other. There are many different versions of color wheels. The first color wheel was invented by Sir Isaac Newton in the mid-1660s.   **p. 5**

Complementary pairs: see *complements.*

Complements: colors directly opposite one another on the color wheel. Complements, also called *complementary pairs* or *contrasting colors,* neutralize one another when combined. Green and red are complements, orange and blue, and so on.   **p. 11**

Concentrates (also called *jewel tones, intensifiers, mixers, modifiers, fortifiers, mixtones, accents, creators, kickers* and so on): the purest, most intense colors in a haircolorist's palette, mixed with other colors to strengthen (intensify) the tone of formulas.   **p. 64**

Configuration: the straightness or curliness of hair, which is an aspect of texture. The shape of the individual hair strands is what makes hair naturally straight, wavy, or curly: the rounder the hair shaft, the straighter the hair; the flatter the hair shaft, the curlier the hair.   **p. 24**

Contrasting colors: see *complements.*

Contrasting formula: a haircoloring formula intended to contrast-out (neutralize) an unwanted tone.   **p. 114**

Contrast-out: to make neutral in tone; to mute the tone of a color by adding its complement.   **p. 10**

Contributing pigment: see *dominant underlying color.*

Cool colors: colors in the range of green-to-blue-to-violet on the color wheel; colors that lack warmth.   **p. 11**

Copper green: green discoloration of hair caused by the absorption of copper in water; also called *chlorine green.* See *swimmer's hair.*   **p. 123**

Corrective haircoloring: haircoloring services performed in order to change existing artificial color.   **p. 98**

Corrective lowlighting: a lowlighting service to correct overlightness, especially overlightness caused by repeated highlighting or excessively heavy highlighting. Corrective lowlighting may be used to add depth to any previously lightened hair.   **p. 118**

Cortex: the second and most substantial layer of the hair strand. The cortex contains nearly all of the melanin of hair, and is also the source of its strength and elasticity.   **p. 16**

Creeping oxidation: continued oxidation; occurs when traces of alkaline material remain in the hair following a bleaching or haircoloring service; causes rapid fadage.   **p. 83**

Cuticle: the protective outer layer of the hair strand, consisting of highly keratinized, overlapping scales. In very dark hair, the cuticle may contain some melanin.   **p. 16**

Cystine bonds: see *disulfide bonds.*

Decolorizing: color-removal service; partial or complete removal of artificial haircoloring. The word *decolorizing* is sometimes used to refer to the lightening of natural pigment as well.   **p. 119**

Decolorizing products: products used to remove artificial haircoloring, also called *color removers.* (The word *decolorizer* is sometimes used to mean *bleach,* any bleaching product.) **p. 119**

Demarcation (line of demarcation): a visible difference between colors on the hair shaft, especially the line between natural outgrowth and artificially colored midshaft. **p. 36**

Demineralizing treatment: a treatment used to remove unwanted mineral deposits from the hair. **p. 123**

Demi-permanent haircoloring: oxidation haircoloring used only to deposit; a deposit-only, no-lift category. Demi-permanents generally fade less dramatically and offer more coverage than do semi-permanent colors, but do not, or should not, lighten natural pigment, unlike permanent haircoloring. **p. 34**

Departmentalization: establishing areas in the salon for different services, such as cutting in one area and coloring in another. A departmentalized salon often has specialized stylists. **p. 142**

Deposit-only haircoloring: haircoloring that only deposits artificial pigment, without lightening natural pigment; also called *no-lift* haircoloring. The term *deposit-only* is used especially in reference to demi-permanent products, but describes any haircoloring product incapable of lifting natural pigment. **p. 34**

Detoxifying products: see *clarifying products.*

Developer ratio: ratio of color to developer, either 1:1 (one to one, equal parts of color and developer) or 1:2 (one to two, one part color to two parts developer). **p. 78**

Developer strength: the concentration of hydrogen peroxide in a developer, expressed in percent or volume. **p. 64**

Direct dyes: dyes that color the hair directly, without developer. Direct dyes are *preformed* and color the hair without an oxidation process, simply staining the cuticle and, to whatever degree they penetrate, the cortex. **p. 34**

Disulfide bonds: sulphur-to-sulphur bonds that cross-link amino acid (polypeptide) chains in the cuticle and cortex of hair. *Disulfide* means *two sulphur atoms;* a *disulfide bond* is a chemical link between two sulphur atoms. Also called *cross, cystine,* or *sulphur bonds.* **p. 17**

Dominant underlying color: the dominant natural color tone underlying a given level of haircolor. Each level of natural haircolor can be said to have one identifiable, dominant tone, which makes that haircolor what it is, in terms of its lightness or depth. Determining a client's natural base level tells you what their dominant underlying color is. Other terms for *dominant underlying color* include *contributing pigment, natural underlying pigment, undertones,* and *residual pigment.* **p. 21**

Double-application: an application method that involves mixing and applying the color formula twice. Usually refers to the double-application method of virgin application, but retouches can be double-application, too. **p. 79**

Double-application method of virgin application: a color application on hair having no existing tint, in which haircoloring is applied twice. Color is first applied ½″ away from the scalp out to the overporous ends and allowed to process 15 minutes or so, then fresh color is mixed and applied to the scalp area and out through the ends. This is the technique of virgin application for high-lift blonds, for bright reds (with permanent haircoloring), and for the most complete coverage of gray. The use of color processing machines may reduce the need for double-application. **p. 79**

Double-process: a color service which involves two haircoloring processes, usually one to lighten and one to tone. *Double-process* usually means *bleach-and-tone.* **p. 96**

Drabbers: ash concentrates, mixed into cool formulas for greater neutralization of natural underlying warmth. **p. 65**

Dye intermediates: tiny, colorless dye molecules that combine when oxidized, forming large, colored molecules. Dye intermediates, also called *dye precursors* must undergo oxidation in order to color hair. Haircoloring containing dye intermediates is oxidation haircoloring, and is mixed with a developer. **p. 39**

Dye precursors: see *dye intermediates.*

Dye sensitization: sensitized to (allergic to) dyes. **p. 77**

Eumelanin: one of the two main types of melanin in hair. Eumelanins are dark pigments, ranging from black to brown. Also see *pheomelanin.* **p. 18**

Eumelanosomes: melanosomes that contain eumelanin. **p. 18**

Existing tint: artificial haircoloring already present in the hair. Existing tint is one of the Five Key Factors that Affect the Haircoloring Result. **p. 49**

Extreme overporosity: extensive damage to the cuticle. Requires adjustment to haircoloring formula or technique. If hair is so damaged that it is breaking off, it should not be colored.

See *abused rejection, overporous hair*, and *porosity.* **p. 26**

Eye color: eye color consists of the dominant color of the iris, but the iris usually also has dashes, bands, and flecks of other colors. Eye color is either warm, cool, or neutral. Eye color may be the deciding factor in selecting a target color. **p. 56**

Fadage: loss of artificial pigment (loss of tone, intensity, or depth) from artificially colored hair that occurs over time as a result of shampooing or other lifestyle or environmental factors. **p. 25**

Fibrils: fibers composed of smaller fibers. The cortex of hair consists of complex, rope-like, protein fibrils, surrounded by a matrix of protein and cross-linked by disulfide (cystine) bonds. These fibrils consist of protofibrils, roped together to form microfibrils, which are roped together to form macrofibrils. **p. 17**

Fine hair: hair that is finer than average (the individual hairs are fine in diameter). Fine hair tends to color more quickly than hair of average texture, and fade more quickly as well. Fine hair has less cortical area than average hair, and more surface area per its unit weight (a high proportion of cuticle). Hair may be fine only in certain areas, most commonly, the hairline. More people think they have fine hair than really do. See *texture.* **p. 24**

Five Key Factors that Affect the Haircoloring Result: the five characteristics of hair that affect the final haircoloring result. The Five Key Factors are natural base level, percentage of gray, texture, porosity, and existing tint. Assessing the Five Key Factors is an integral part of the Universal Method of Formulation. **p. 46**

Follicle: the tiny pocket, or sheath, in the skin that houses the hair root. **p. 16**

Formulating: determining what formula will achieve the target color; deciding what you have to put on the client's hair to produce the desired color result, given her key factors (natural level, percentage of gray, texture, porosity, and whether there is any existing haircoloring). **p. 64**

Gray hair: naturally unpigmented, or nearly unpigmented, hair. The terms *gray hair* and *white hair,* while technically different, are used interchangeably in this book and by most stylists. Technically, completely unpigmented hair is actually white in appearance and hair that appears gray contains a minute amount of pigment; for formulation purposes, however, the two are the same. See *percentage of gray* and *white hair.* **p. 24**

Hair bulb: the live part of a hair strand, at the base of the hair root, from which the hair grows. **p. 16**

Hair root: the part of a strand of hair which is below the surface of the skin. **p. 16**

Hair shaft: the part of a strand of hair which is above the surface of the skin. **p. 16**

Henna: a form of botanical, or vegetable, haircoloring; consists of a dry powder that is mixed with hot water to form a nonoxidizing, no-lift dye paste. Henna is extracted from the bush of the same name, which is native to India, Egypt, and the Middle and Far East. Professional hennas may be compounded with other plant dyes. Unlike professional products, hennas sold for home use may be compounded with metallic dyes. **p. 37**

High-lift tint: haircoloring intended to lift more than two levels; permanent haircoloring

using more than the standard (usually 20 volume) developer. **p. 26**

Highlighting: a haircoloring service to lighten selected strands within a head of hair. The word *highlighting* usually refers to foil highlighting, or another enclosure method of highlighting (highlighting papers, for instance), but can also mean cap highlighting (using a frosting cap) or any creative highlighting technique. Highlighting may be done with one formula or multiple formulas, with bleach or permanent haircoloring, all over or in a single area. A touch-up highlighting is a highlighting on the new growth only. The word *highlighting* covers a lot of territory; techniques are many, as are the color effects produced. **p. 91**

Holiday: a euphemism for bright spots or streaks at the scalp area when foils or frosting caps bleed. **p. 111**

Hue: see *tone.*

Hydrogen peroxide: a compound of hydrogen and oxygen (H_2O_2) used as an oxidizing and bleaching agent. Hydrogen peroxide is the oxidizer (developer) of oxidation haircoloring (demi-permanent and permanent haircoloring products). **p. 39**

Hyperpigmentation: increased melanin production (darkening of the hair); associated with certain illnesses or drugs. **p. 125**

Hypopigmentation: decreased melanin production (whitening of the hair); associated with certain illnesses or drugs. **p. 125**

Indirect dyes: dyes that must undergo oxidation in order to color hair. The aniline-derived dye intermediates of demi-permanent and permanent haircoloring are indirect dyes.

Haircoloring that contains indirect dyes is mixed with a developer. **p. 35**

Infrared lights: heat-producing lamps, used to accelerate haircoloring processes. **p. 83**

Intensity: see *tonal intensity.*

International Level System: see *Universal Level System.*

Keratin: a tough, fibrous, high-sulphur protein. Hair is 90 to 95 percent keratin. **p. 16**

Keratinization: the process by which amino acids are converted to keratin. **p. 16**

Keratinized: converted to keratin. **p. 16**

Level: the darkness or lightness of natural or artificial haircolor, indicated by a number. Levels are exact, visually distinct measurements of darkness or lightness, numbered from 0 or 1, to 10 or higher. See *Universal Level System.* **p. 6**

Level-on-level toning: regarding application of color to previously colored or lightened hair, level-on-level means applying a color formula the same level as the current color level of the hair, in order to alter the tone. Here are two examples: 1) Hair prelightened to yellow is toned with a 9 level light blond formula; yellow is the dominant underlying color of a 9 level light blond, and a 9 level formula provides level-on-level toning. 2) A client is recolored with a cool 7 level dark blond formula after blond haircoloring lifted her to an undesirable orange-gold; a 7 level dark blond formula is chosen to contrast-out the unwanted warmth because light orange is the dominant undertone of 7 level dark blond hair. **p. 92**

Light: radiant energy, which travels in waves of varying lengths. White light is all of the wavelengths combined. Color results from the separation of wavelengths, the splitting of white light. **p. 4**

Lowlighting: a haircoloring service to deepen selected strands within a head of hair, done with foil, cap, or in any other way. Lowlighting may be done on a colored head of hair to add dimension and depth (shading), on a gray or graying client to reduce the amount of gray (gray reduction or marbleizing), or to correct excessive highlighting (corrective lowlighting). **p. 91**

Luminosity: how much light a color reflects. Light colors and bright colors reflect more light than do dark colors and muted colors. **p. 9**

Marketing: the practice of identifying consumers' needs and meeting those needs, for a price. **p. 130**

Matrix: the protein in which cortical fibrils are embedded. (**Matrix** can also refer to the germinal region of the hair bulb.) **p. 17**

Medulla: the innermost layer of the hair strand, which is sometimes intermittent or even absent. The medulla may contain some melanin. **p. 17**

Melanin: the pigment that gives human hair its natural color; also occurs in human skin and eyes, as well as in other animals and in certain plants. **p. 16**

Melanocytes: cells that manufacture melanin; hair melanin is manufactured by melanocytes in the hair bulb. **p. 16**

Melanoprotein: protein in which melanin is encased. **p. 18**

Melanosomes: structures in hair, skin, and eyes that store melanin. The suffix *-some* means *body;* melanosomes are melanin-containing bodies. **p. 18**

Metallic dyes: dyes, such as lead acetate, which are derived from metals. Metallic dyes are not used professionally, mainly because of their incompatability with oxidation processes. **p. 37**

Metatoulenediamine: a common aniline derivative dye. **p. 39**

Midshaft: the middle part of the hair shaft; not the scalp area, or warm zone, and not the ends. **p. 28**

Missing primary: the primary color absent from a mixture, which, when added, will result in a neutral tone. When all three primaries are mixed, a neutral tone is created (brown, black, or grey). For example, green (which is blue and yellow) is neutralized by red, its missing primary. **p. 12**

Moderate overporosity: medium overporosity; moderate damage to the cuticle. May require adjustment in haircoloring formula or technique. See *abused rejection, overporosity,* and *porosity.* **p. 26**

Monoethanolamine (MEA): a common ammonia substitute, used to elevate the pH of haircoloring in the same way and for the same purpose as ammonia. MEA is a compound of nitrogen, hydrogen, carbon, and oxygen. **p. 38**

Multiporous: having different degrees of porosity down the length of the hair shaft. See *porosity.* **p. 28**

Multi-shading: a highlighting and/or lowlighting service using two or more formulas, usually done with foil or highlighting papers. The word *shading* implies deepening, but *multi-shading* has come to mean multiple formulas, whether lighter or darker than the base color. **p. 54**

Munsell Sphere: a three-dimensional model of a color circle that graphs hue, level, and tonal intensity; invented by early 20th century American painter Albert Munsell. **p. 8**

Natural base level: how light or dark hair is naturally, also called *natural level, natural base,* and *base level.* Natural base level is one of the Five Key Factors that Affect the Haircoloring Result. **p. 46**

Natural contribution of the hair: see *dominant underlying color.*

Natural underlying pigment: see *dominant underlying color.*

Neutralize: to make neutral in tone or pH. To neutralize a color means to mute it or contrast it out by coloring over it with its complement, which produces a neutral tone, neither cool nor warm. To neutralize alkalinity means to bring the pH to a neutral state, which is 7, that of distilled water. **p. 10**

No-lift haircoloring: haircoloring that does not lighten natural pigment, also called *deposit- only haircoloring.* Temporary and semi-permanent haircoloring, as well as color-and-shine glazes, are incapable of lightening and so are no-lift products. Demi-permanents are generally no-lift as well. **p. 35**

Nonoxidizing: substances that do not oxidize; colorants that do not undergo an oxidation process in order to color hair (direct dyes).

Temporary and semi-permanent haircoloring, as well as color-and-shine glazes, are nonoxidizing. **p. 76**

Normal porosity: describes hair that has a slightly raised cuticle. Slight ruffling is normal, because everything hair is exposed to (shampooing, styling, sunlight, and so forth) has a weathering effect. Normal hair is neither resistant nor damaged in appearance. See *porosity.* **p. 26**

Off-the-scalp techniques: application techniques that do not involve placing haircoloring directly on the scalp. Foil highlighting is an off-the-scalp technique. **p. 76**

1:20 test: a test for metallic salts in hair. *1:20* refers to the ratio of clear 20 volume hydrogen peroxide *(one ounce)* to household ammonia *(twenty drops)* that makes up the test liquid. A sample of hair is dropped into the test liquid and observed for reactivity. **p. 120**

Opaque: blocking light. Opaque haircoloring doesn't allow light to filter through the strands. Haircoloring done with an opaque product looks dense, solid, and heavily or uniformly colored. Contrast *translucent.* **p. 48**

Overacceptance: absorption of more artificial pigment than normal. See *overporous hair.* **p. 26**

Overporous hair: hair with a raised and eroded cuticle, which makes it look damaged and feel rough. Overporous hair accepts haircoloring faster than normal, selectively absorbs ash dyes, and fades sooner than normal. See *abused rejection, extreme overporosity, moderate overporosity, normal porosity, porosity.* **p. 26**

Overtoning: see *browning-out.*

Oxidation (oxidative) haircoloring: haircoloring that must undergo an oxidation process in order to color hair. Oxidation haircoloring is mixed with a developer. Demi-permanent and permanent haircoloring are oxidative products. **p. 35**

Oxidize: to combine with oxygen. When melanin is lightened with hydrogen peroxide, which is an *oxidizer,* it is *oxidized,* or combined with and broken apart by oxygen, which is a chemical change. When the artificial pigments of oxidation haircoloring are mixed with hydrogen peroxide, they also are oxidized and chemically reformed. **p. 35**

Oxymelanin: partly oxidized melanin. **p. 21**

Paper charts: printed charts that color companies provide to display the colors of haircoloring systems. **p. 47**

Papilla: the tiny mound of tissue beneath the hair bulb, interlaced with capillaries that nourish the growing hair. **p. 16**

Paraaminophenol: a common aniline derivative dye. **p. 39**

Paraphenylenediamine (PPD): the most commonly used aniline derivative dye. **p. 39**

Paratoulenediamine: a common aniline derivative dye. **p. 39**

Patch test: see *predisposition test.*

Penetrating tint: an obsolete term for permanent haircoloring, originally given this name because of its ability to fully penetrate the hairshaft. **p. 37**

Percent of hydrogen peroxide: a measure of the strength of a hydrogen peroxide developer; the concentration of hydrogen peroxide in water. For example, a 3 percent solution of hydrogen peroxide, which is the same as 10 volume, contains 3 percent hydrogen peroxide and 97 percent water. **p. 36**

Percentage of gray: the amount of gray; the ratio of unpigmented to pigmented hair in a client's natural base. For example, 10 percent gray means that 10 out of 100 hairs is gray. Percentage of gray is one of the Five Key Factors that Affect a Haircoloring Result. **p. 48**

Permanent haircoloring: haircoloring products capable of lightening natural pigment and designed to permanently alter natural haircolor. All products in this category are oxidative, using aniline derivative dyes and hydrogen peroxide developers. (Hennas and metallic dyes, because they don't fade quickly, were once considered permanent haircoloring, but are no longer categorized as such.) **p. 37**

Personal selling: your personal recommendation; recommending services and products to clients. **p. 133**

pH: a measure of the acidity or alkalinity of aqueous (water-containing) solutions. Values run from 0 to 14; 7 represents neutrality, numbers less than 7 represent increasing acidity, and numbers greater than 7 represent increasing alkalinity. **p. 38**

Pheomelanin: one of the two main types of melanin in hair; pheomelanins are medium to light pigments, ranging from red-brown to red-yellow to yellow. Also see *eumelanin*. **p. 18**

Pheomelanosomes: melanosomes that contain pheomelanin. **p. 18**

Pigmented shampoos and conditioners: shampoos and conditioners that also deposit color; such products are temporary or semi-temporary haircoloring. **p. 95**

Pigmented styling and finishing products: styling and finishing products (gels, mousses, sprays, and pomades) that also deposit color; such products are temporary or semi-temporary haircoloring. **p. 32**

Pigments: chemicals in living and nonliving things that give those things color by modifying light, absorbing some wavelengths of light and reflecting others. The part of light that is reflected is what we perceive as color. **p. 4**

Porosity: the ability of hair to absorb and retain moisture, determined by how raised or compact the cuticle layers are; commonly referred to as *condition*. Porosity, which is described as resistant, normal, or overporous, is one of the Five Key Factors that Affect a Haircoloring Result. **p. 25**

Positioning: image-building, which is an aspect of marketing; establishing in your clients' minds, or in the public's mind, what kind of place your business is. **p. 130**

Predisposition test: a test for dye sensitivity (allergy to haircoloring), performed on a patch of the client's skin prior to a haircoloring service; also called a *sensitivity test* or *patch test*. **p. 77**

Preformed dyes: see *direct dyes*.

Preshampooing: to shampoo the hair immediately before application of haircoloring so that the color is applied to clean, and usually damp, hair. Preshampooing is gentle, without manipulating the scalp, followed by gentle, thorough towel-blotting. **p. 81**

Primary colors: the first colors, from which all other colors are derived. The three primary pigments are red, yellow, and blue. **p. 10**

Principle of light and dark, the: light extends or maximizes; dark recedes or minimizes. Lighter, more luminous colors are more prominent visually; they advance, enlarge, and appear more airy. Darker, less reflective colors recede; they appear farther away, smaller, and more dense. This is the art principle that color contouring is based upon. **p. 58**

Professionalism: conduct, appearance, and personal qualities that assure clients of your expertise and ethics. **p. 131**

Promotion, promotional activity: any business activity designed to creatively inform your clients or potential clients what it is you have for sale and to enhance the reputation of your business. **p. 130**

Promotional mix: the combination of promotions you undertake, how you blend different forms of promotional activity. **p. 133**

Protinator: another name for the booster packet (activator) mixed into scalp bleach. **p. 96**

Reducing agents: substances that cause reduction reactions, which are the opposite of oxidation reactions. The action of permanent wave solution is an example of a reduction reaction; ammonium thioglycolate and thioglycolic acid are reducing agents. Oxidation haircoloring may be removed with a decolorizer containing a reducing agent, followed by an oxidizer, but this type of decolorizer is much less commonly used than bleach removers. **p. 119**

Reflectivity: see *luminosity.*

Residual pigment: see *dominant underlying color.*

Resistant hair: hair that has a compact cuticle which resists absorption, also termed *tenacious*

hair. Resistant hair is slick and glossy, more difficult to penetrate than average hair, and can be said to have *"poor porosity."* See *porosity.* **p. 26**

Retouch application: haircoloring application to the new growth on color-treated hair. **p. 79**

Reverse-frost: a lowlighting service done with a frosting cap (the hair pulled through the cap is deepened rather than lightened), especially to deepen previously frosted hair, but for other effects, too (to disguise gray, for instance). **p. 119**

Scalp-to-ends: application of haircoloring from the scalp to the ends; often the technique for virgin application and, particularly with no-lift haircoloring, sometimes the technique for retouch. **p. 79**

Scalp-to-ends virgin application: a first-time application (no existing tint) in which haircoloring is applied from the scalp to the ends. This is the method of virgin application for demi-permanent haircoloring, and for matching or going deeper than the natural level with permanent haircoloring. Semi-permanent haircoloring and color-and-shine glosses are also applied this way, except bright or deep formulas, which are applied just barely off-scalp (application to only the hair, not the scalp, to avoid staining the scalp). **p. 79**

Secondary colors: the colors immediately derived from the primary colors, resulting from the combination of two primaries. The three secondary pigments are orange, violet, and green. **p. 10**

Semi-permanent haircoloring: no-lift haircoloring that lasts approximately haircut to haircut, gradually fading over a period of about four weeks. Semi-permanents are direct dye stains, are not mixed with developers, and are incapable of lightening natural pigment. **p. 34**

Semi-temporary haircoloring: products that have characteristics of both temporary and semi-permanent haircoloring.   **p. 33**

Sensitivity test: see *predisposition test.*

Shade system: a system of categorizing artificial haircoloring by *shade,* which simply means *variation in color*, rather than identifying colors by level and tone.   **p. 8**

Single-process: a color service involving only one haircoloring process; usually refers specifically to permanent haircoloring.   **p. 91**

Skin stain remover: a product designed to remove haircoloring stains from the skin, the main ingredient of which is often isopropyl alcohol.   **p. 83**

Skin tone: the underlying hue of skin. Skin has either warm or cool undertones, visible in skin of any lightness or depth. Skin with yellow or orange undertones is considered warm; cool skin has blue-pink or blue-red undertones. Skin tone is often the most important consideration in selecting a target color; in general, warm haircoloring enhances warm skin, cool haircoloring enhances cool skin.   **p. 56**

Smaller- and higher-weight dyes: small and large dye molecules.   **p. 35**

Specialization: to choose a speciality, such as cutting or coloring.   **p. 142**

Soapcap: obsolete term for *emulsifying color through the ends;* a technique to gently refresh color on overporous ends during a retouch, by diluting leftover haircoloring or color already on the hair with water, then lathering the ends

with it. Sometimes shampoo is added, but color chemistry is such now that water is more often used.   **p. 80**

Sodium bromate: a chemical occasionally used in the neutralizer of permanent waves. The active ingredient in the neutralizer of almost all professional permanent waves is hydrogen peroxide, but hydrogen peroxide reacts with metals, so if hair has been colored with metallic dye, a sodium bromate neutralizer is recommended.   **p. 105**

Solvents: substances that other substances will dissove in. Examples of common solvents include water, isopropyl alcohol, and mineral or castor oil.   **p. 119**

Steamers: warm mist machines, used to accelerate haircoloring processes.   **p. 83**

Strand test: usually means a *preliminary* strand test, in which a small amount of the color formula is mixed and applied to a finger-thick strand, in order to test the effectiveness of the formula *before* the complete application. Cleaning and looking at a strand of hair while the color processes may also be called a strand test.   **p. 77**

Stripper, stripping the hair: obsolete terms for *color remover, color removal.*   **p. 119**

Surface-acting: affecting only the surface of the hair shaft; not penetrating. Temporary haircoloring products are surface-acting.   **p. 32**

Swimmer's hair: hair characterized by chlorine and copper damage (swelling and abrasion of the cuticle; glassy, coated feel; greenish cast visible on hair that is light brown or lighter). **p. 105**

Synthetic swatches: swatches of synthetic hair provided by manufacturers to display the colors of their haircoloring systems. Synthetic fibers are used because they retain color better than does natural hair. **p. 47**

Target level: the level that you are trying to achieve in a given haircoloring service; the desired level. **p. 24**

Target market, target clientele: the people you want your business to serve. **p. 130**

Temporary haircoloring: haircoloring that lasts shampoo to shampoo, the color deposit washes out completely or almost completely in a single shampoo; temporary haircoloring is surface-acting, not penetrating, and incapable of lightening natural pigment. This category includes temporary rinses, pigmented shampoos and conditioners, pigmented styling and finishing products, and various other forms (crayons, mascaras, powders, and so on). **p. 32**

Tertiary colors: the third colors *(tertiary* means *third)*, produced by combining a primary color and one of the secondary colors next to it on the color wheel (red with violet, for instance). The six tertiary pigments are red-violet, red-orange, yellow-orange, yellow-green, blue-green, and blue-violet. **p. 11**

Texture: the diameter of the hair strands, either fine, medium (average), or coarse. The greater the diameter of the hair shaft, the coarser the hair; the less the diameter, the finer the hair. Texture, in this sense, is one of the Five Key Factors that Affect a Haircoloring Result. The word *texture* also refers to the configuration of hair—straight, wavy, or curly—as well as to the general feel of hair, which is a function of diameter, configuration, and condition. **p. 24**

Tint-back (tinting-back): a haircoloring service to darken previously lightened hair, restoring it to or near its natural depth. Tinting-back often requires prepigmenting (filling). **p. 117**

Tonal intensity: the strength, or purity, of a tone. The most intense colors are the most pure. Colors that are less intense are adulterated with other hues. **p. 8**

Tonal series: a succession of levels of artificial haircoloring having a common tone. **p. 7**

Tone: hue; the hue of natural or artificial haircolor. The main tones of haircolor are neutral (natural), ash, gold, and red. **p. 7**

Total coverage: completely colored; every strand tinted, no gray remaining. **p. 65**

Translucent: permitting light to pass through. Translucent haircoloring allows light to diffuse through the strands, allows the eye to see "into" the hair, and so has a somewhat dimensional appearance (appears to have top-tones and undertones). Contrast *opaque.* **p. 36**

Tricochromes: a type of natural pigment that occurs in some red hair. Tricochromes are yellow-red pigments found especially in carrot-red hair. **p. 19**

Underacceptance: absorbing less artificial pigment than normal. See *resistant hair.* **p. 26**

Undertones: see *dominant underlying color.*

Universal Level System: a system of categorizing natural and artificial haircolor by levels of lightness or darkness, using numbers to indicate level, from 1 (darkest) to 10 (lightest). **p. 6**

Universal Method of Formulation: the method of formulation that applies to all types and brands of haircoloring products, consisting of careful communication, analysis of all factors that will affect the final color result, and determining a specific target color, before mixing color.   **p. 6**

Virgin application: haircoloring application on hair that has not been colored before (hair that has no artificial color already on it). **p. 79**

Volume: a measure of the strength of a hydrogen peroxide developer; the amount of oxygen a given concentration of hydrogen peroxide will release. For example, 10 volume hydrogen peroxide (H_2O_2), which is the same as 3 percent, releases 10 times its volume in oxygen (one ounce of 10 volume H_2O_2 releases ten ounces of oxygen). 20 volume H_2O_2 releases 20 times its volume (two ounces of 20 volume releases 40 ounces of oxygen). **p. 38**

Warm colors: colors in the range of yellow-to-orange-to-red on the color wheel.   **p. 11**

Warm zone: the first quarter-inch of hair next to the scalp, also simply called the *scalp area,* which has the benefit of body heat during haircoloring processes.   **p. 80**

White hair: naturally unpigmented hair. When the hair bulb stops producing melanin, hair appears white. See *gray hair.*   **p. 88**

Working volume: refers to the volume strength of a developer-and-color or developer-and-water mixture. For example, a formula of 1 part color and 1 part 10 volume H_2O_2 has a working volume of 5. A formula of 1 part color, 1 part 10 volume H_2O_2, and 1 part distilled water has a working volume of 3.33 (3⅓). Haircoloring mixed with equal developer has a lower working volume than haircoloring mixed with double developer. **p. 115**